IMMUNIZATION
IN CLINICAL PRACTICE

edited by
VINCENT A. FULGINITI, M.D.
Professor and Head
Department of Pediatrics
College of Medicine
University of Arizona

five contributors

IMMUNIZATION
IN CLINICAL PRACTICE

*A Useful Guideline to Vaccines, Sera, and
Immune Globulins in Clinical Practice*

J.B. Lippincott Company • *Philadelphia* • *Toronto*

The authors and publisher have exerted every effort to ensure that drug selection and dosage set forth in this text are in accord with current recommendations and practice at the time of publication. However, in view of ongoing research, changes in government regulations, and the constant flow of information relating to drug therapy and drug reactions, the reader is urged to check the package insert for each drug for any change in indications and dosage and for added warnings and precautions. This is particularly important when the recommended agent is a new or infrequently employed drug.

Copyright © 1982, by J. B. Lippincott Company.
All rights reserved. No part of this book may be used or reproduced in any manner whatsoever without written permission except in the case of brief quotations embodied in critical articles and reviews.
For information address J. B. Lippincott Company, East Washington Square, Philadelphia, Pennsylvania 19105.

1 3 5 6 4 2

Library of Congress Cataloging in Publication Data

Main entry under title:

Immunization in clinical practice.

Includes bibliographies and index.
1. Immunization. I. Fulginiti, Vincent A.
[DNLM: 1. Biological products — Therapeutic use.
2. Immunization. QW 800 I32]
RA638.I53   615'.37   81-8314
ISBN 0-397-50539-6   AACR2

Printed in the United States of America

This volume is dedicated to
C. HENRY KEMPE, M.D.,
former Professor and Chairman of the
Department of Pediatrics,
University of Colorado, School of Medicine.
His labors are appreciated by the
entire pediatric community and,
to an even greater degree,
by the children whose lives he has touched,
both directly and indirectly.

Contributors

E. Russell Alexander, M.D.

Professor and Head
Section of Infectious Diseases
Department of Pediatrics
College of Medicine
University of Arizona

Vincent A. Fulginiti, M.D.

Professor and Head
Department of Pediatrics
College of Medicine
University of Arizona

H. Robert Harrison, D.PHIL., M.D., M.P.H.

Assistant Professor
Department of Pediatrics
College of Medicine
University of Arizona

James F. Jones, M.D.

Assistant Professor
Department of Pediatrics
College of Medicine
University of Arizona

C. George Ray, M.D.

Professor, Pediatrics and Pathology
Director, Virus Diagnostic Laboratory
Arizona Health Sciences Center
University of Arizona

Contents

4. PRACTICAL ASPECTS OF IMMUNIZATION PRACTICE

Vincent A. Fulginiti

5. THE SCHEDULING OF IMMUNIZATIONS

Vincent A. Fulginiti

6. DIPHTHERIA
C. George Ray

7. PERTUSSIS
Vincent A. Fulginiti

Preface

Successful immunization practice is one of the most important activities in total comprehensive care for children. Pediatricians, family practitioners, general practitioners, nurse practitioners, school physicians, school nurses, public health practitioners, and others may be involved in the art and science of immunization. This book was prepared because the person involved in immunization practice needs a single source for complete information concerning practical immunology, vaccines, and antibody preparations.

If one seeks information concerning the rationale, safety, and efficacy of immunizing biologics, one encounters numerous resources. Standard textbooks, specialty texts, national and local advisory group publications, and the medical literature may need to be consulted in order to pin down a single answer to a specific question in practice. Even with these numerous sources, the answers to some questions are in places so obscure or difficult to locate that the seeker never obtains them. This is evidenced by the abundant number of queries from practitioners which are directed to consultants, advisory groups, health departments, and other authoritative sources. The authors, having observed this phenomenon in the last two decades, thought that a single reference source might prove useful as a repository for answers to many of the common, repetitive questions that occur in everyday practice. This volume was born from such a conception.

We organized, developed, and wrote this text with the practice of immunization in mind. Hence, we have opted for a narrative style without heavy reference insertions in the text in order to make it easily readable. References are appended to each chapter and include both classic and recent literature and other citations. These are selected to allow an interested reader to dig more deeply into specific issues, if desired.

The text has enough theoretic background to enable the reader to grasp underlying concepts inherent in the recommendations. Both historic and futuristic sections are included to enable us to see how we got here and where we are going. The bulk of the text is devoted to where we are, with specific disease sections for all vaccines and biologics likely to be encountered in practice.

Of necessity, there is much judgment and opinion included. For many practical questions of vaccine and antibody usage, there are no specific data to guide us. In such areas, the authors and editor have selected one or more options from among those available for consideration. The reader is advised that these are *judgments* and are clearly indicated as such in the text.

Each author has written the chapters under his name. However, the editor has liberally reviewed each and revised them (1) to update information as close to the time of delivery of the manuscript to the publisher as possible; (2) to achieve consistency in content from section to section; (3) to add illustrative material, in some instances; and (4) to satisfy his personal style for certain expressions of ideas, concepts, or facts.

Several of the contributors have been, or are, members and consultants to local, regional, and national advisory groups, including the American Academy of Pediatrics Committee on Infectious Disease, the Advisory Committee on Immunization Practice of the Center for Disease Control and the writing committee for the American Public Health Association's publication, *Control of Communicable Diseases.* As a result, many of the recommendations are similar to, or almost identical with, portions of documents these members wrote for such bodies. In some instances, precision in recommendations was deemed so important that the language used, of necessity, mimics that found elsewhere. The purpose is to avoid ambiguity in circumstances where exact recommendations need to be offered.

Finally, it is essential for everyone to recognize the dynamic nature of immunization theory and practice. What is true today is false tomorrow, and *vice versa.* This phenomenon is particularly evident in areas where judgment has been exercised because of paucity of data or lack of information. The editor was vividly reminded of this phenomenon when he received a letter from a friendly critic contrasting a published opinion given in 1963 with one written in 1980 on the same subject. The opinions were diametrically opposed, the change occurring as a result of investigational and experiential data in the intervening 17 years!

Our knowledge of immunology, virology, and the interactions between the two is at times fragmentary and tentative. But we do learn and we can modify both our thoughts and our practices. Flexibility, and not rigidity, is the watchword of immunization theory and practice. Utilization of this principle has enabled medicine to move forward with elimination and diminution in the toll of infectious diseases as the reward for mankind.

—Vincent A. Fulginiti, M.D.

Acknowledgements

We are indebted to our secretarial staff who responded to our sometimes insistent, unreasonable, and insatiable requests for typing, retyping and re-retyping. Of particular note are the contributions made by Jo Anne Jenkins from the inception to completion of the project. The final manuscript was organized and typed by Cheryl Czaplicki who introduced us to the marvels of electronic typing and editing. Others whose efforts are appreciated include Suzanne Levy, Dorothy Bates, Linda Minnich, and Betty Noriega.

Finally, we could not have accomplished this task without the cooperation and understanding of our spouses and children.

1
History and Overview

Vincent A. Fulginiti

THE EARLY HISTORY OF IMMUNIZATION

Man has attempted to prevent nature's ravages since the dawn of history. Even before the infectious nature of disease was appreciated, empiric observations led intelligent men to surmise a cause–effect relationship between a disease and the abnormal material that developed in the affected person, and a primitive concept of transmissibility developed. Dixon, in his excellent text on smallpox, cites its being known as a discrete disease as early as 1160 B.C. It is likely that the disease existed since antiquity but this is the first recorded description.

Ramses V, Pharoah of Egypt, apparently had the disease, as evidenced by his mummified remains. In the Tcheou Dynasty of China (1122 B.C.), smallpox was called "tai-tou." The Chinese first utilized inoculation as early as 590 B.C. by implanting bamboo splinters dipped in pustular material into the nasal mucosa of uninfected individuals.

A Sanskrit text, *Saetaya*, presents evidence of variolation in India centuries before Christ. Such early attempts appear to have been shrouded in magic and superstition, often with mystical and religious overtones: hence, the concept that one could transfer the pestilence from the affected individual to an animal or another human, thereby releasing an evil spirit from the sick person.

This mystical characteristic, plus an erratic use of the practice, had no practical influence upon the epidemiology of smallpox. Such impact awaited a clearer definition of transmissibility and the accumulation of empiric observations before a systematic approach could be attempted. Hence, Jenner's epochal vaccination of James Phipps was preceded by common wisdom, which described the transmissibility of the disease and the preventative characteristics of mild illness. Apparently, a num-

1

ber of unknown individuals appreciated the fact that the natural transmission of smallpox, such as to a nursing mother from an infected infant, resulted in mild disease in the mother and protection in case of future contact. Also, farmers knew that the disease, cowpox, was associated with lesions on the udders of cows which, when handled, often gave rise to similar lesions on the hands of the milker. A further link was provided with the observation that milkers so afflicted either did not get smallpox, or if afflicted, had a milder, nonlethal form of the disease.

Jenner synthesized these observations and performed his classic experiments from which the origins of modern immunization stem. He was not the first to prevent smallpox; rather, his contribution was to substitute an inoculous local infection, cowpox or vaccinia, for smallpox. For centuries before Jenner, the practice of variolation was known and pursued, and actual smallpox material was transferred from one patient to another, often by means of an infectious scab. Although successful in some, variolation had the hazard of occasionally producing full-blown disease in the susceptible person. On rare occasion, death occurred as a result of such transfer.

Vaccination changed the odds and made the transfer of the related agent, vaccinia virus, safer and more predictable. After Jenner, our history is rich in anecdote of the trials and tribulations of vaccination and variolation. Reading these accounts, one recognizes the full spectrum of human triumph and foible. Vaccination became a medical, political, religious, ethical, and social phenomenon, often simultaneously. Not until the advent of modern biologic knowledge did the procedure and its descendents assume a more balanced place in human history. Scientific and medical considerations became uppermost, although all the other human factors continued to play a role, albeit in a subdued fashion. Even today, religious, ethical, and political considerations tinge our practices to some extent and are explored in Chapters 3 and 25.

THE MIDDLE PERIOD OF IMMUNIZATION HISTORY

The first scientific attempts to prevent natural disease occurred as a result of Pasteur's experiments with veterinary diseases. Aged cultures of attenuated fowl cholera and anthrax bacilli were used to immunize susceptible animals. In both instances, these animals became remarkably resistant to challenge by virulent organisms. In parallel and in sequence, other investigators explored the use of killed and attenuated bacteria in the prevention of human disease. Koch discovered cell-mediated immunity during a search for a vaccine to prevent tuberculosis. Von Behring and Kitasato discovered diphtheria antitoxin and passive immunity during primitive studies of diphtheria immunization.

In 1884, Solomon and Smith demonstrated that killed hog cholera bacillus (a salmonella) protected pigeons against virulent challenge. In 1896, Pfieffer and Cole immunized two humans with heat-killed typhoid bacilli. Almrath Wright drew on these two events to develop an effective typhoid vaccine in 1898. At that time, typhoid was more devastating than war. It killed 5,000 people each year in England and 35,000 each year in the United States. The case fatality rate ranged from 10% to 30%; seven times as many soldiers died from typhoid as from battle injuries in the Spanish–American War.

Wright systematically tested a heat-killed typhoid vaccine until 4,000 Indian Army volunteers had received it. Reactions to the vaccine were severe, but protection was striking; the mortality rate decreased from 14% to 2%. Despite problems with politics and excessive vaccine reactivity, additional large-scale studies were carried out during World War I. Among 1,125,000 immunized British troops, only 7,500 cases of typhoid occurred with 266 deaths. In contrast, during the South African War, 73,633 unimmunized soldiers contracted typhoid and 10,144 died. This early success encouraged others to explore the use of cholera and plague vaccines, and opened the door to modern bacterial vaccinology.

Reactions to all of the bacterial vaccines were severe but protection against disease was striking. Despite the reactions and despite technologic accidents resulting in virulent or contaminated vaccines, progress continued and culminated in the development of vaccines against diphtheria, tetanus, pertussis, and other bacterial diseases. For a full review of this fascinating area in microbiology and medicine in human history, the reader is recommended to the books by Parish.

THE MODERN PERIOD OF IMMUNIZATION HISTORY

Although some view the progress in immunization as a long, continuous thread involving the development of scientific thought and investigative microbiology, several events stand out as major determinants of rapid progress.

Pasteur, in 1884, was the first to modify a virus by serial passage in another species. He developed so-called fixed rabies virus which distinguished the attenuated agent from the natural "street" virus. Pasteur passaged rabies virus in rabbits and, after more than 100 passages, the fixed virus had little capacity to infect dogs when given subcutaneously. Pasteur extracted the spinal cords of infected rabbits at this high passage level and dried them at room temperature. He then gave ten daily subcutaneous injections and discovered that dogs were made resistent to experimental infection when an appropriate dose was used.

In 1885, a peasant boy who had been severely bitten by a rabid dog came to Pasteur's attention. He was to be the first human to be immunized against rabies using the same method developed for dogs. Pasteur theorized that the long incubation period of rabies in humans would allow development of immunity by vaccine stimulation. The treatment appeared to work and the child remained well. Information about this immunizing procedure rapidly became known, and Pasteur and other individuals began to use fixed virus to protect against rabid exposure in humans.

Thus, by the end of the 19th century and the beginning of the 20th, a large number of individuals had begun experimenting with both live and killed infectious agents in an attempt to substitute an immunizing experience for the natural disease. Although many anecdotes could be told about these attempts, those connected with influenza are most instructive for our purposes. Pandemics and epidemics of influenza were recognized as far back as the early 1500s. In the latter part of the 19th century, there were 55 years in which influenza was epidemic in various parts of the world. Major pandemics with horrible morbidity occurred during the 18th and 19th centuries.

The modern era and influenza immunology began with the isolation of the influenza virus by Smith and co-workers in 1933. (Previously, influenza was thought to be a bacterial disease and was attributed to *Hemophilus influenza*.) They were also able to demonstrate that convalescent sera from patients who had had influenza contained neutralizing antibody to the virus. We now know that this was influenza type A, and repeated outbreaks occurred in the early 20th century.

A long period followed up to the present time in which various antigenic changes of influenza type A were observed and described, and influenza viruses types B and C were isolated and identified, and shown to be different antigenically from type A. During this period, it was discovered that recovery from infection was accompanied by antibody development, and that in experimental animals, antibody production and immunity appeared to be equated. Further, injection of active or inactive virus in such animals, by routes other than the respiratory system, resulted in the development of circulating antibody and resistance to natural challenge.

Field studies in the early part of the 20th century gave inconsistent results. Often, the disease had a low natural incidence, and the potency and antigenic composition of vaccines were not equated with the then current epidemic strains. In 1943, the Army conducted a classic study employing controls and clearly demonstrated that immunization with concentrated formalin-inactivated influenza viruses prepared from embryonated hens' eggs prevented epidemic influenza with an effectiveness rate of greater than 75%. Since that time, extensive technologic improvement and expansion in our epidemiologic and virologic information have permitted a wide variety of influenza vaccines to be developed, tested, and proven effective. Greater details as to current immunology concerning the influenza virus are given in Chapter 16.

Enders, Weller, and Robbins' Nobel Prize winning work in 1949 established the methodology whereby modern virus vaccines were developed. Their contribution was the discovery that polioviruses could be cultivated *in vitro* in primate tissue of nonnervous tissue origin. Prior to that time, all viral vaccines were developed in animals or in embryonated hens' eggs. Such vaccines were necessarily crude and many contained host-derived materials or active virus, which had markedly adverse effects upon the recipient. A brief exploration of these efforts is warranted.

In the 1930s, poliovirus vaccines were prepared from the spinal cords of infected monkeys. In retrospect, only type 2 virus was included. The vaccines were inactivated with phenol or ricinoleate. Those efforts failed. In some instances, fully active poliovirus was administered, with devastating results. In one trial, paralytic polio developed in ten of 10,725 recipients after the first or second dose. At this time, it was not known that three types of poliovirus existed and that nonparalytic infection also occurred.

Just prior to the discovery made by Ender and colleagues, scientists were sorting out the biology and classification of poliovirus and delineating the full infectious spectrum. These efforts laid the biologic and epidemiologic foundations for the development and deployment of vaccines derived from tissue culture methods.

Jonas Salk prepared formalin-inactivated poliovirus vaccines for each of the three types by repeated passage in monkey kidney tissue cultures. In 1954, following small-scale trials that established antigenicity and safety, the massive Francis Field Trial was undertaken in the United States. Unequivocal efficacy and safety was demonstrated and the vaccine was licensed in 1955. There was one setback, the Cutter incident, involving large amounts of administered vaccine in which inactivation of poliovirus was incomplete, resulting in paralytic disease in some recipients. More stringent manufacturing and safety testing guidelines were developed, and the vaccine was widely used with a resultant sharp decrease in poliomyelitis.

In 1952, the first safe live polio virus vaccines prepared in simian tissue culture were administered to humans by Koprowski and colleagues. Over the next five years, three separate sets of candidate vaccine strains were developed by Koprowski and colleagues, by Cox and co-workers, and by the Sabin group. The Sabin vaccines were selected for massive use, and after their field trials and introduction commercially, they gradually replaced inactivated (Salk) vaccine.

In 1954, Enders and colleagues isolated measles virus from a 14-year-old with the surname Edmonston. From this isolate were derived two isolate strains, one of which became adapted to chick embryo tissue culture after passage in human tissue culture and fertile hens' eggs. This development opened the current era of live virus immunization, with similar techniques being employed for preparation of live rubella, mumps, and varicella vaccines, among others, and for sufficient growth of rabies virus to permit production of highly antigenic inactivated vaccine.

The remarkable progress made since 1949 can be traced directly to the epochal observations of Enders, Weller, and Robbins with poliovirus. Added to the tissue culture technology are today's use of virus fractionation (to produce subunit vaccine in highly purified and concentrated form), ultracentrifugation (to produce concentrated products in large quantities), and other technologic improvements in vaccine manufacture.

The final contribution in the modern era was the cultivation *in vitro* of human diploid fetal cells by Hayflick and Moorehead in 1961. These cell strains retained the normal chromosome number (diploidy) and could be serially maintained *in vitro* for a sufficient period to achieve huge masses of cells. At first blush, such cell strains might be considered ideal for vaccine production, because the hazards of antigens from other species being incorporated into vaccines are avoided. However, it took more than a decade from their discovery to vaccine utilization. Of primary concern was whether unknown, potentially disease-producing agents might be present in such tissue. It was feared, on theoretic grounds alone, that transfer of a latent agent might result in deleterious effects such as cancer or chronic neurologic disease many years later. However, a sufficient body of observation in human volunteers receiving vaccines prepared in human fetal cells and exhaustive laboratory attempts to uncover latent agents has resulted in assurance that such risks apparently do not exist.

As a result, at least three currently used common vaccines are prepared in human diploid fetal cells: inactivated rabies vaccine, oral live poliovirus vaccine, and live rubella virus vaccine.

We have not seen the end of a viral vaccine technologic triumph. Some enthusiasts visualize a future replete with safe viral vaccines for most common and some uncommon diseases. Some of these speculations, as well as realistic prospects for the more immediate future, are included in Chapter 25.

Work in bacterial vaccinology did not go undone during this period of intense virologic investigation. A number of attempts have been made to refine and purify bacterial components responsible for eliciting immune responses in humans, but progress has been considerably slower than in virologic investigation. Some components of bacteria have been clearly identified as having the characteristics necessary to afford protection. For example, the current pneumococcal vaccine is derived from the polysaccharide capsule of the organism and is a noninfectious chemical constituent capable of evoking a sufficient serum antibody response to be protective in some persons against challenge with the pneumococcal types from which the polysaccharides are derived. Similar preparations have been manufactured for the meningococcus and for *Hemophilus influenza* type B. However, success has been more limited than that encountered with pneumoccal polysaccharide. These diseases are discussed more fully in subsequent chapters.

Bacteriologists have also attempted to develop attenuated strains of bacteria that might be administered orally and afford protection against diseases such as shigellosis and cholera. These efforts are more fully discussed in Chapter 25.

ANALYSIS OF IMMUNIZATION HISTORY

The history of immunization has spanned relatively few decades in the entire history of mankind. Despite this temporal limitation, significant advances have been made in our understanding of the pathogenesis of disease and in the immunologic response of the host, which permits startling changes in the epidemiology of disease. We have seen smallpox completely eliminated from the world and major decreases in pertussis, diphtheria, poliomyelitis, measles, and other contagious diseases. Furthermore, we have learned how to provide specific protection against diseases such as tetanus by using a specific product of a bacterium to induce a specific immune response. Overall, the health of mankind, and particularly of children, has benefited; classic morbidity and mortality experienced in early life as a result of infectious diseases have been reduced or eliminated.

However, we have not eliminated all problems associated with infection control. In fact, we have created some new ones, and have been remarkably unsuccessful in dealing with some old problems. On balance, though, we should view our accomplishments with considerable pride inasmuch as we have appeared capable of discerning major natural threats to our well-being and of devising methods for the control or elimination of these threats. There are still major gaps in our knowledge of infectious disease virulence, in the pathogenesis of many illnesses, and in the immunologic responsiveness against a variety of infectious antigens. We can only anticipate that improved scientific methods will continue to overcome these barriers, and that more efficient products will emerge and be used in prevention.

However, we must not forget the political and social issues still encountered in immunization theory and practice. We have not solved many issues involving the application of specific vaccines, the balance between safety and efficacy, the ability to estimate and evaluate theoretic long-term risks, and similar issues in the deployment of effective and available products. We will discuss some of these issues in Chapters 2, 3, 4, and 25, but a brief presentation here seems appropriate.

Technologically, we appear more capable of identifying agents responsible for disease, isolating them in some *in vitro* system, and bottling them as antigens, than we are in deciding upon their use. Varicella virus will serve as an example here. Using the principles developed since Enders' original discovery and applying them to measles, rubella, mumps, and other agents, Japanese workers have isolated an attenuated varicella virus in a human diploid tissue culture system. They have begun cautious experimentation with this product and have had remarkable success thus far.

In the United States, an active debate has ensued concerning whether varicella vaccine of this type could be employed. The major point of dispute is centered on the biologic properties of varicella virus, or more properly, on our ignorance of some of the biologic properties of varicella virus. We know, for example, that natural varicella virus infection results in an acute infectious disease of which the manifestations are usually self-limiting and mild. However, the virus does not disappear from the body but remains dormant within sensory ganglia of the nervous system. Occasionally, it emerges and produces herpes zoster in some individuals. The mechanisms behind this latency phenomenon are obscure and ill-defined. Nevertheless, many virologists believe it is a universal phenomenon in all individuals exposed to varicella virus.

The reactivation of varicella virus from its latent site in such disease states as leukemia and lymphoma, or following the administration of certain chemotherapeutic agents or ionizing radiation, has resulted in severe disease with predictable mortality. In addition to our lack of understanding of latency and reactivation, we also are incapacitated by the lack of uniformly effective treatment for such severe disease.

In this context, varicella virus vaccine in attenuated form has not been adequately studied for its potential to produce latency, nor has enough time elapsed to indicate whether reactivation will occur at all, and if it occurs, whether it will be a major problem. On the one extreme, some individuals argue that we may expect to see a large number of instances of herpes zoster occurring as a result of attentuation of the virus (which *might* enhance its capacity to become latent). On the other hand, proponents of varicella vaccine argue that no such evidence exists and that the risk is theoretic at best. There are all shades of opinions between these two extremes.

As a result, we are uncertain today, in the United States, whether or not varicella vaccine should be employed as a routine immunization in childhood; rather, a very cautious investigative approach has been undertaken of using it in the highest risk group, namely, those children who are in remission from leukemia and who are found to be susceptible to varicella. This group has been investigated by the Japanese, and the vaccine has been found to be safe and effective in evoking an immune response and protection from subsequent challenge. For the time being, this will be the level of investigative effort in the United States, and until the issue of the theoretic and actual risks of latency are resolved, further use of the vaccine in a routine fashion is unlikely. Similar arguments are developing for and against the use of vaccines prepared from other DNA viruses of the herpes group, cytomegalovirus and *Herpes hominis*.

The foregoing is an example of scientific uncertainty conditioning investigation and use of a particular vaccine. In addition, we have numerous social considerations that influence the deployment of some vaccines, for example, some argue that universal reimmunization with rubella vaccine is desirable. For reasons that will be apparent by reading Chapter 9 on rubella, not all humans are immune and it is unlikely that standard routine programs of rubella immunization will reach the entire population. As a result, it has been recommended that rubella vaccine be administered uniformly to all prepubertal children in school in an effort to achieve near-100% immunization. I will not explore the theoretic arguments against this practice here (they are detailed in Chap. 9), but will highlight the social issues involved.

Health-care dollars in the United States are limited and cannot be garnered in sufficient amounts to do everything we desire. If it were practical to reimmunize universally against rubella, this effort would require an enormous expenditure of public funds to accomplish its objective. It would also be expensive in terms of health-care-worker time and effort. Since funds and resources are limited, undertaking reimmunization would necessitate diminishing some other health-care activities. At present, we are incapable of resolving this issue in our society, and as a result, the public health sector is unwilling to consider such a practice further, since it believes it will interfere with other goals in immunization and public health that are equally vital and productive.

Finally, religious and other personal considerations sometimes preclude the individual's acceptance of immunization. We have religious groups and cults that object to the administration of vaccines to their children, even if such objection is in violation of statute or regulation. This results in social conflict that is difficult to resolve, because we respect both the religious and other rights of individuals to determine their own fate while at the same time that we hold dear the right of society at large to be protected against contagious diseases. This is a difficult issue to resolve if we attempt to preserve both the individual's and society's rights (see Chap. 3 for fuller discussion).

Further muddying the water are issues of liability. Many vaccine products have intrinsic risks associated with the biologics they contain. Such risks result in a predictable morbidity and even mortality when the product is given to millions of recipients. Our society's tradition is that individuals have a right to seek redress in a court of law when damage has been done as a result of some intrinsic defect in a product that they use. In the case of immunizations, the risk may be a natural biologic activity of the infectious agent, and the damage either the result of a disease induced by or some side-effect or toxicity of the product. In recent years, legal activity against manufacturers, government agencies, individual physicians, hospitals, clinics, and a host of other individuals and institutions has been taken as a result of such adverse consequences of vaccine administration. We have not yet resolved, as a society, who should assume liability, and we do not have a uniform system for determining the cause, effect, and extent of liability. Thus, individual legal action carried through our tort law system often determines how such issues are resolved, so that individual court decisions can have an impact upon the practice of immunizations. This topic is dealt with more fully in Chapter 3.

Thus, scientific advance is not sufficient to determine the fate of individual immunization efforts. Even if we assume adequate immunologic and infectious disease knowledge, and the capacity to produce an effective biologic agent, we must still overcome political, social, and other issues influencing the use of such products in a complex and highly individualistic society such as ours.

REFERENCES

Bean JA, Burmeister LF, Paule CL, Isacson, P: A comparison of national infection and immunization estimates for measles and rubella. Am J Public Health 68:1214–1216, 1978

Dixon CW: Smallpox. London, Churchill Ltd., 1962

Dudgeon JA: Immunization in times ancient and modern. J Royal Soc Med 73:581–586, 1980

Horstmann D: Viral vaccines and their way. Rev Infect Dis 1:502–516, 1979

Madoff MA, Gleckman RA: Immunizations, where the money should be. J Infect Dis 133:230–232, 1976

Monto AS, Ross HW: Swine influenza vaccine program in the community, reactions and responses. Am J Public Health 69:233–237, 1979

Parish HJ: A History of Immunization. Edinburgh, E & S Livingstone, 1965

Parish HJ: Victory with Vaccines. Edinburgh, E & S Livingstone, 1968

Wilson G: Hazards of Immunization. London, Anthalone Press, 1967

2

Immunology of Immunization

James F. Jones
Vincent A. Fulginiti

Administration of a vaccine is intended to elicit an active response in the host, such that on natural exposure to the infectious agent, the host resists infection. Inherent in this concept is the complex interaction between the host and the immunizing agent. An understanding of host defense mechanisms responsible for protection against the various types of infectious agents and of the components or products of the causative agent responsible for an individual disease is imperative for development, administration, and evaluation of vaccines.

The development of tetanus toxoid is an example. At least two requirements had to be met before this vaccine could have been conceived and produced: (1) identification of the toxin produced by *Clostridium tetani* which caused the disease and (2) determination that antitoxin antibody protects the immune host from the effects of the disease-producing toxin. Development of a safe, effective vaccine available for wide distribution followed successful efforts to alter the toxin, rendering it safe and yet immunogenic. Once produced, indications for its use and the timing of administration of primary and booster doses ensured appropriate duration of protective circulating antibody levels. Antecedent to these steps was the development of assays to measure the immune response derived from basic immunologic investigation.

In this chapter, the active and passive immunization principles inherent in vaccine development are reviewed. With a more comprehensive understanding of these principles, the practitioner may better appreciate the advantages and limitations of vaccines, antisera, and immune globulins.

OVERVIEW OF THE IMMUNE SYSTEM AS IT RESPONDS TO A NEWLY INTRODUCED CHALLENGE

The response of an organism to infection is multifactorial; an example will serve to illustrate the complex interactions of various *host* components.

A pathogen is inhaled and adheres to and enters pharyngeal lymphoid tissue. The infectious agent becomes engulfed by fixed phagocytic cells or macrophages which may kill and digest the pathogen. Alternatively, the agent may replicate without host interference. In either case, the macrophage "processes" the pathogen and is able to pass on information about the invader to other cells. Communication with other cells, B and T lymphocytes, requires recognition by the cells of each other and of the pathogen. These cell–cell interactions are under genetic control and information is probably transmitted by RNA.

Antigen may bind directly to B lymphocytes with appropriate receptors on their surfaces. These cells proliferate and mature into antibody-producing plasma cells manufacturing specific antibody directed against the various antigens of the pathogen. This is the *primary response.* Other specific B lymphocytes become memory cells and circulate or reside in organized lymphoid tissue. The memory cells respond to another challenge by the same organism through rapid proliferation and heightened manufacture of antibody (the *secondary response*).

For some pathogens, the macrophage interacts with T lymphocytes which have specific receptors for the pathogen and for the macrophage. Once T lymphocytes are triggered by the macrophage–pathogen complex, they proliferate as did the B lymphocytes, and at least five subsets of cells result: memory cells, lymphokine or mediator-producing cells, helper cells, suppressor cells, and killer T cells. The mediators include macrophage inhibitory factor (MIF), neutrophil chemotactic factor, interferon, and many others. These chemicals produce and participate in the inflammatory response. T helper cells enhance the production of antibody by stimulating activated B lymphocytes; T suppressor cells inhibit antibody and lymphokine production. This serves to modulate the response. Specifically activated T killer cells recognize the pathogen directly or recognize its presence in or on the membrane of infected cells and lyse the agent or infected cell.

Complex interactions among these cells and their products, if effective, limit and remove the offending agent. In addition, lasting protection or immunity develops as a result of memory cell stimulation. This protection prevents reinfection with the specific agent and other pathogens that are similar antigenically.

It is this recall or protective function of the immune system that we depend upon in active immunization. By eliminating natural infection and substituting an innocuous exposure to an agent or its antigen, we bypass the harmful effects of the infection but stimulate the host just as if infection has actually occurred. Both characteristics of the pathogen and the host determine the type, extent, and efficacy of the immune response.

Characteristics of the Pathogen

All microorganisms have complex and varied structures. The components of pathogens that the host recognizes are termed *antigens* or *immunogens*. Antigens may be of varying types: protein, polysaccharide, lipid, or nucleic acids. For the purposes of preparing vaccines, proteins and polysaccharides are most important as they are most antigenic.

Of basic importance to the development of immunity is the "foreignness" of antigens. Immunologic response is geared to recognition of antigens that the host does not possess. Another important characteristic of an antigen is its size; most large molecules are good antigens. However, large polysaccharide molecules with repeating sugar moieties are poor antigens. Complex substances with molecular weight of over 100 to 1500 daltons are usually considered of adequate size to stimulate an immune response. However, large molecules, (>100,000 mw) are more immunogenic than small ones.

The structure of an antigen is also important. Antibodies may be formed against the primary (amino acid sequence), secondary (backbone or polypeptide sequence), tertiary (folding or confirmation of the molecule), or quaternary (multiple subunits) structure of a protein molecule. Complexity of an antigen correlates well with its immunogenecity. The portions of the antigen molecule that trigger a reaction and actually combine with antibodies or receptors on T lymphocytes are termed *antigenic determinants*. Thus, specific, complex portions of antigen molecules more readily stimulate an immune response.

The potency of the immune response to antigenic determinants is controlled by the accessibility of antigenic determinants. The terminal side-chains of polysaccharides and the most exposed amino acid sequence of polypeptides are most immunopotent. The tertiary structure or conformation of the molecule determines accessibility by the degree to which these terminal sequences are exposed to host cell surfaces.

Haptens differ from larger antigens in that if used alone to inoculate an animal, little if any immune responses (particularly antibodies) are elicited. If a hapten is covalently coupled to a protein carrier, however, specific antibodies are produced after injection into experimental animals or humans.

Factors Affecting Immunogenicity of Antigens

Native protein is usually a better immunogen than material that has been heated or treated with enzymes. However, it is necessary to alter natural protein to reduce its toxic or disease-producing effects while preserving its antigenicity. Formaldehyde treatment, for example, removes biologic activity but doesn't alter immunogenecity of molecules such as diphtheria and tetanus toxin and of more complex antigens such as pertussis bacilli.

Dose size affects the quantity, affinity (strength of binding to antigen), and specificity of antigens; low doses enhance each of these characteristics. Application of this concept to humans is difficult because each antigen varies in induction of immune response and a sufficient dose must be employed to develop any response. Polysaccharide and live, attenuated viruses are particularly dose-dependent.

The route of administration of a given antigen governs the type of response. Parenteral administration assures rapid contact with regional lymphoid tissue and is effective in evoking antibodies against a variety of agents. In natural disease, such agents tend to spread their toxic products through the circulatory system and adequate levels of circulating immunoglobulin, that is, tetanus and diphtheria toxins, will prevent disease manifestation. Administration of killed polio vaccines also gives adequate serum levels of antibody and protects against systemic spread of the virus (see Chap. 12).

Administration of other vaccines by the "route of natural infection," that is, salmonella, cholera, shigella, and *E. coli* (currently under investigation), is based on the principle of inducing local as well as systemic immune responses in hopes of inducing more complete immunity. Oral polio vaccine is based on this principle in that ingested virus both induces a local IgA response in the gut and evokes systemic antibody production. This serves to provide a barrier to infection as well as to prevent systemic spread should infection occur.

Efforts to enhance immunogenecity include mixing of antigens with a variety of adjuvants or substances that augment the immune response. The principles behind such efforts include: delay of antigen destruction, increase of antigen dispersion, and increase of lymphocyte traffic to lymph nodes sequestering the antigen. Freund mixed antigen with mineral oil and an emulsifier to augment the immune response. This had limited success, but when *Mycobacteria tuberculosis* was added to the mixture (complete Freund's adjuvant—CFA), there was a marked response. In animals, this latter maneuver was eventually shown to enhance response to antigens that require the help of T cells. Thus, CFA modifies the immunoglobulin class produced (IgG versus IgM), overcomes tolerance, and also favors a cell-mediated response. However, it cannot be used in humans, and other adjuvants have been sought.

Mineral salts, such as aluminum hydroxide, have been used extensively to enhance antibody production (*e.g.*, tetanus toxoid). Inclusion of these salts in vaccines induces local granuloma formation, which inhibits dispersion and allows deposits of antigen needed for primary and secondary responses to develop in sequence. In theory, alum-precipitated material is needed only for the first injection, as it adds nothing when used in subsequent injections in the same individual. Practice and convenience, however, preclude change of vaccines, and the adjuvant vaccine is usually the only product available.

Host Factors That Affect the Immune Response

Specific genetic makeup will determine the quantity and quality of host–immune response. Recognition of the antigen, rate of synthesis of antibody, and the type of immune response are all under genetic control. Investigation in this area is primitive, but valuable clues are rapidly being uncovered.

In the first place, the host must recognize the antigen as foreign. To do so, a mechanism for recognition of "self" or host antigens must be present. Man appears to have an elaborate self-recognition system, partially based on chromosome number 6 in the so-called HLA region.

This genetic locus determines the antigens that stud the surface of host cells—providing a type of "fingerprint" at the cellular level. The normal host is genetically incapable of mounting an immune response against such antigens.

There are two consequences of this system: (1) antigens similar to the host antigens are not responded to; and (2) antigens dissimilar from the host evoke an immunologic reaction. For example, variola virus has some antigens that resemble or are identical to group A substances on human erythrocytes. Evidence from population studies suggests that smallpox may be more prevalent among humans with blood type A than among humans with other blood types.

Most pathogens have an antigenic structure that is sufficiently different from human cell antigens that they are all recognized as foreign. This appears to occur because of the presence of the human immune response (Ir) genes located in or near the HLA locus. These genes direct the synthesis of immunoglobulins in some fashion, determining the capacity of the host to respond.

Individuals with certain HLA types respond differently to infectious antigens than do individuals with other HLA types. Most information in this area has been gleaned by investigation of a similar system in mice (H-2 system). Pure-bred mice with precise definition of H-2 type can be bred to react with no, some, or a great deal of antibody to specific antigens. Their response appears to be directly related to their H-2 "fingerprint."

Observations concerning humans are more indirect, and no populations analogous to pure-bred colonies of mice exist. What has been noticed is that individuals with differing HLA types respond to antigens, such as that of influenza virus, to different degrees. Some individuals are low responders, that is, they produce small amounts of antiinfluenza antibodies when given killed influenza vaccine. Others are medium responders and some are high responders. The degree of response has been related to possession or lack of specific HLA antigens. Our current knowledge of this phenomenon is scant, but it appears to be an important factor in determining the immune response.

Other genetic loci determine the degree of host–cell interaction. If one recalls that the type and briskness of the response to infectious agents is partially dependent upon cell-to-cell communication, then it is apparent that genetic variability in the interaction will influence immunity.

One example will serve to illustrate this phenomenon. In the HLA region, there is a locus that determines the presence or absence of an antigen (Ia) on immune cell surfaces. The degree to which macrophages that have ingested an infectious agent communicate information about the antigen of that agent to lymphocytes is partially dependent on the presence of Ia antigens on each of the cell surfaces. Thus, the character and function of the Ia gene may determine the capacity of lymphocyte response and control of such immune functions as T-cell activation and proliferation and, hence, modulation of the total response.

It is certain that even more complex genetic control exists. Certain phenomena remain unexplained. For example, males, in general, are more susceptible to most infections and suffer greater mortality than do females. Whether this is a result of a lack of one X chromosome, or due to some specific characteristic of Y chromosome function, or both, or neither, we simply do not know.

The unraveling of genetic immunologic control offers a promising avenue for future investigation. For the present, we must recognize that individuals vary in their immunologic capacity, and vaccine evaluation must take these phenomena into account.

Synthesis

Interaction between T and B cells and the concept of hapten-carrier protein molecules as antigens has previously been cited. These phenomena are interwoven in host response to certain antigens, as follows.

Repeating sugars in chains, polysaccharides, may be recognized by B cells in the absence of thymocytes. The response may be production of antigen-specific IgM or induction of tolerance, a state in which no overt immune response occurs. If this polysaccharide is covalently coupled to a protein molecule, a hapten-carrier molecule is formed. When this combination is administered to a genetically responsive host, IgM and then IgG antibodies are produced, a process that requires T helper cells in conjunction with B lymphocytes. In this case, B lymphocytes appear to have receptors for the hapten (polysaccharide) and T lymphocytes appear to have receptors for the carrier molecule, and in order to produce IgG antibodies or cell-mediated immunity (CMI), both cell types must be present and in communication with one another.

Production of antibodies against lipids and nucleic acids also requires coupling of these types of antigens to carrier protein molecules.

Polysaccharide antigens and some polymerized protein antigens are referred to as thymus-independent antigens. As described, these molecules may interact with B lymphocytes directly and form IgM antibodies; although this reaction is possible, a biologic purpose is not yet apparent.

Many questions concerning the host's response to antigens remained unanswered, not the least of which is why some antigens evoke primarily an antibody response and why others produce CMI. Qualitative or quantitative differences in immunogenecity do not account for this apparent dichotomy of response. In fact, the separation may be more apparent than real, and we may have measured only one aspect of the host's response when several are taking place and are necessary for the development of immunity.

Measurement of the Immune Response to Immunization

Clinical and laboratory methods are available for measuring natural or acquired (after immunization) immunity. Specific antibodies against diphtheria toxin can be detected by means of the Schick test. A small amount of toxin is injected intradermally; if antibodies are present, no reaction is seen.

A positive skin test is detectable if delayed hypersensitivity to an antigen is present (*e.g., M. tuberculosis*).

These *in vivo* tests have been used for years but have several disadvantages; they are not quantifiable and are dependent upon observation that may be faulty. Recent attempts have been made to measure immune responses *in vitro*.

The majority of laboratory assays available are for detection of a specific antibody. A complete discussion of methodology for detection of antibodies is beyond the scope of this chapter. We will concentrate on the most frequently used tests in determining response to immunization.

Each test uses the specific interaction between antigen and antibody

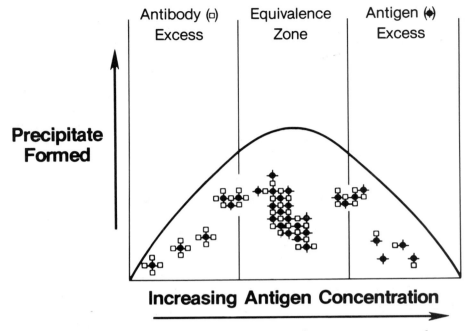

Fig. 2-1. The relationship of antigen/antibody concentrations to formation of precipitate.

to detect the presence of antibody; the tests differ in the physical form of the antigen that is used. If the antigen is soluble, both components may diffuse through a suitable medium and a visible precipitate is formed where they interact. By modifying the concentration of the components, a quantitative assay is produced (Fig. 2-1).

Thus, the results of the test are highly dependent on the conditions under which it is performed. Antibody levels seen in the equivalence zone are most closely associated with the expected biologic activity (*i.e.,* opsonization or toxin neutralization). In addition, soluble immune complex (antibody–antigen complexes in antigen excess) are associated with a variety of clinical illness (serum sickness, acute glomerulonephritis, etc.).

Precipitation reactions (gel diffusion, immunoelectrophoresis, and radial immunodiffusion) are most useful in quantifying immunoglobulins or in qualitatively analyzing abnormal immunoglobulin molecules in a variety of disease states. Their relative insensitivity in quantitation of specific antimicrobial antibodies precludes their usefulness in these assays (see Table 2-1).

Similar chemical principles govern agglutination reactions, a very

TABLE 2-1. Sensitivity of Quantitative Tests Measuring Antibody Nitrogen of High-Avidity Antibody

Test	mg Ab N/ml or Test
Precipitin reactions	3–20
Immunoelectrophoresis	3–20
Double diffusion in agar gel	0.2–1.0
Complement fixation	0.01–0.1
Radial immunodiffusion	0.008–0.025
Bacterial agglutination	0.01
Hemolysis	0.001–0.03
Passive hemagglutination	0.005
Passive cutaneous anaphylaxis	0.003
Antitoxin neutralization	0.003
Antigen-combining globulin technique (Farr)	0.0001–0.001
Radioimmunoassay	0.0001–0.001
Enzyme-linked assays	0.0001–0.001
Virus neutralization	0.00001–0.0001
Bactericidal test	0.00001–0.0001

common means of assaying specific antibody production. In these situations, the antigen is adsorbed to solid particles, that is, erythrocytes and biologically inert materials, such as, latex beads, and the end-point is a readily visible clumping of the particles. In antibody excess, no clumping is seen as in the precipitation reaction; however, because particles are present, no decrease in the reaction is observed in the antigen excess zone. The agglutination reaction is more sensitive because the lattice formed between antigen and antibody is visibly enhanced by the particles, whereas in the precipitation reaction, a huge amount of antibody is required to form a visible lattice.

Agglutination reactions can be performed directly or indirectly. When the antigen in question is a component of the particle used in the assay (*e.g.*, bacteria) addition of specific antibody will cause direct clumping. Soluble antigen may adhere spontaneously to red blood cells or may be chemically linked to other particles, and thus can serve as a tool for indirect measurement of antibodies.

Care must be exercised in judging responses to this test, as antibody excess may preclude formation of an appropriate lattice. This problem is obviated by dilution of serum specimens. IgM is more likely to form a lattice (because of its pentameric structure), and, therefore, care in timing of samples is important in judging the results of this assay. For instance, use of thymus-independent antigens (*i.e.*, pneumococcal polysaccharide) may induce IgM antibodies detectable at 2 weeks, but will not induce lasting protection because IgG antibodies are not produced.

Another property of immunoglobulin useful in quantitating specific antibody is its ability to fix complement. The assay depends upon activation of complement by sheep red blood cells coated with anti-sheep-erythrocyte antibodies with an end-point of lysis of the erythrocytes. In the first stage of the test, patient serum is added to test serum in the presence of a known amount of guinea pig complement. The second stage is initiated by the addition of the sensitized sheep erythrocytes. If specific antibody to test antigen is present in the serum sample, complement will fix, and hence, no complement is available for hemolysis of sensitized red blood cells.

Neutralization of pathogens themselves is a very sensitive assay for specific antibodies and is believed to be most representative of immunity. Quantitation of antiviral (*e.g.*, antipoliovirus) antibodies is particularly useful and sensitive. Test sera are diluted and added to tissue culture, egg, or animal systems, and inhibition of virus replication or effect is determined. Dilution of test sera allows a titer to be determined as in each of the other assays.

More recently, a variety of other assays with increasing sensitivities have been developed. Instead of directly measuring antibody–antigen interactions, as in the precipitin–agglutination reactions, these newer techniques take advantage of a further component of immunoglobulins—their own antigenicity. In these assays, test serum is added to a variety of solid materials which contain the antigen in question. After allowing an antigen–antibody reaction to occur, a labeled (histochemical or radio-) antiimmunoglobulin produced in rabbits or goats is added to the system. Dilution of the test serum allows titration of the response if the label is fluorescent or if color changes and an +/− reaction is visualized; or the label may be quantitated giving an indirect, but highly sensitive and reproducible, measurement of specific antibody.

Thus, a variety of antibodies may be detected to indicate an immune response to antigen(s) of a particular infectious agent. Such examinations have a number of clinical uses. They can be used for detection of the immune status of an individual patient to assist in determining the need for an immunization; *e.g.*, rubella virus antibody in a female. They can be used for population surveys to detect adequacy of protection as needed for immunization efforts for a particular disease and to determine immune status if a hazard to immunization exists (*e.g.*, measles antibody level in a patient with leukemia). On occasion, they can be used to monitor the efficiency of a given immunization procedure in practice.

All such determinations are limited by the biologic significance of the detectable antibody. For example, parainfluenza virus vaccines were administered experimentally to children and evoked detectable serum hemagglutination–inhibition antibody, but little or no neutralizing antibody. The children were unprotected on subsequent challenge. The detection of serum antibody in killed measles virus vaccine recipients was unassociated with protection; in fact, such individuals were at increased risk for development of a severe, atypical form of measles.

In addition to antibody assay, there are assays under development for CMI response to specific agents. These are not clinically useful at present. All depend upon antigen interaction *in vitro* with lymphocytes from immunized or naturally infected individuals.

Performance of these assays is usually not available at the local level because the need arises infrequently. If the practitioner perceives such a need, consultation with state health departments or the CDC should be undertaken. At various medical schools and large hospitals, experts are usually available to assist in this effort.

PASSIVE IMMUNIZATION

In contrast to active immunization, passive transfer of preformed antibody provides almost immediate but short-lived protection against some infectious diseases. In this section, the general principles of passive immunization are reviewed. Specific products and uses are discussed in Chapters 23 and 24.

THE RATIONALE FOR PASSIVE IMMUNIZATION

As discussed earlier, the presence of circulating specific antibody is responsible for "immunity." This means that certain infectious agents or their products exert their disease-producing potential by circulation and distribution through the bloodstream. If antibody is present in the circulation, it may combine with the responsible antigens and inhibit or ameliorate their effect.

In a susceptible host who has been exposed to and is incubating certain infections, the provision of specific antibody may halt the progression to disease. Certain factors are necessary if this effect is to be achieved. (1) The infectious agent or its products must be susceptible to neutralization by antibody. (2) The antibody administered must be of the appropriate type to neutralize the infectious agent or its product(s). (3) The amount of the correct antibody must be sufficient to achieve the desired neutralization. (4) The antibody must be delivered in time to exert its effect. (5) The side-effects of antibody administration must not exceed the consequences of the disease against which protection is sought.

Not all infectious agents are influenced by antibody. Those that are may be variably affected. For example, hepatitis virus A may still produce infection despite passive administration of specific antibody; the disease is prevented but infection is not. On the other hand, measles virus is completely neutralized and neither infection nor disease results if specific antibody is passively administered under appropriate conditions, as will be discussed.

Passive antibody does not prevent or ameliorate pertussis. This is probably due to a combination of factors, including inaccessibility of the organism in the respiratory tract to circulating antibody of the IgG type. Harder to understand is the inefficacy of passively administered mumps antibody; in this disease, one might expect prevention because the virus is neutralizable *in vitro* by antibody. However, data for clinical effect are lacking and passive antibody for mumps is no longer recommended or available.

The specific type and activity of antibody may determine its efficiency. If a low-avidity IgM antibody is given, it may not neutralize an agent that is principally affected by high-avidity IgG.

The amount of the antibody in the preparation used (concentration) and the amount given (dose) also influence the final effect. For example, rubella-neutralizing antibody is present in such low titers in most human immune serum globulin, that even large or massive doses do not provide protection against the disease.

Antibody can only be effective prior to some critical stage in infection. After this point is reached for a specific agent and disease, administration is no longer effective. For example, one must give measles antibody within the first few days after exposure. Beyond this point, the disease occurs irrespective of the presence of antibody. This is a complex phenomenon specific both for the disease and the host. Such factors as the rate of multiplication of the agent, its fixation onto and entry into cells which conceal it from antibody, and the distribution, both in rate and concentration of antibody, will determine outcome in a given clinical situation.

Finally, the disease burden must be weighed against any side-effects of the antibody preparation used. For human-origin antibody, this consideration is almost always unimportant. For antibody contained in animal serum, it may become the determining factor in use or nonuse of such preparations. For example, one may wish to prevent tetanus in a susceptible individual, but horse serum sensitivity may result in anaphylaxis. Therefore, one chooses human antibody without significant risk, although it is more expensive.

CHARACTERISTICS OF PASSIVE ANTIBODY PREPARATIONS

There are two principle types of passive antibody for use in humans: (1) gamma globulin preparations and (2) serum or plasma of either human or animal origin. The characteristics of each are simultaneously similar and different.

Gamma globulin is now officially termed *immune globulin* (IG). In the past, it has been called "immune serum globulin," "human immune globulin," "normal human serum globulin," and other such terms. Today, gamma globulin is prepared from human plasma selected from hepatitis-B-negative donors.

IG is separated and concentrated by the Cohn alcohol fractionation method resulting in a restricted group of serum proteins, principally in the gamma range of electrophoretic mobility. The principle component is IgG, comprising 95% or more of all protein. There are only trace amounts of IgA and IgM and other human proteins.

IG is highly concentrated—a 16.5 ±g/dl solution. The separation and concentration process removes any hepatitis virus that might be present, and the resultant preparation is sterile. It can only be administered intramuscularly since it is strongly anticomplementary. Inadvertent intravenous administration has resulted in anaphylaxis. This is believed to be secondary to the aggregation of IgG molecules that occurs with storage and standing of this highly concentrated solution.

The IgG component contains all four subclasses of IgG (types 1–4) because it is pooled from a large population of humans. Similarly, all genetic types are likely to be present (Gm groups). IgG has a half-life of ±28 days.

Less than 5% of the protein in IG is IgM and IgA, amounts which are insignificant therapeutically with the average half-life of five to seven days of these molecules. No benefit can be expected from the administration of IgM or IgA in the form of IG. IG should be considered to be IgG administration alone in terms of therapy, but the presence of IgA does present possible antigenic stimulation to a recipient who selectively lacks this component in his or her own plasma.

IG should be administered by the deep intramuscular route only. Intradermal administration has no place in therapy or prophylaxis. Subcutaneous injection can be extremely irritating due to the high concentration of protein in IG. Intravenous use of standard IG is contraindicated because of the risk of anaphylactic reactions. In Europe, intravenous preparations have been developed and tested from time to time. There is one such preparation undergoing clinical trial at present. However, there is no commercially available gamma globulin for intravenous use.

When injected intramuscularly, IG must be placed deep in an adequate muscle mass. In general no more than 5 ml should be given at any one site and no more than 15 to 20 ml at any one sitting. It is rarely necessary to exceed 15 to 20 ml as a total dose, even for adults (see Chap. 23).

Serious side-effects of IG are uncommon. Most patients experience some discomfort at the site of injection, often related to the total dose needed.

One final consideration is the high cost of IG, which must be considered in marginal indications.

In one large-scale study, almost 20% of the patients receiving IG had some mild to moderate reactions. These ranged from vague systemic complaints such as nausea and malaise to full-blown anaphylaxis with flushed faces, edema, cyanosis, and collapse. Such reactions were more frequent among former recipients of IG. In our experience, patients in long-term therapy may experience such reactions soon after administration, often of mild to moderate degree, and transient. In some instances, we have been able to link reactions with anti-IgA antibodies in selectively IgA-deficient patients.

In such circumstances, it may be necessary to substitute human plasma from a single donor as outlined below.

CHARACTERISTICS OF SERUM- AND PLASMA-PASSIVE ANTIBODY PREPARATIONS

Various animals can be immunized with specific antigens and large amounts of specific antibody evoked. Serum is then prepared at an appropriate interval and is available for passive prophylaxis.

Animal serum consists of the entire range of subcellular constituents including all proteins. The desired components are the specific antibodies contained in all classes of immunoglobulin molecules. These preparations are standardized to some extent, such that they contain a fixed amount of specific antibody activity as measured against an external standard. For example, diphtheria antitoxin is actually horse serum containing 1,000, 10,000, 20,000, or 40,000 units of antitoxin activity per fixed volume as dispensed. Also, antirabies serum is a refined and concentrated horse serum containing 1,000 U.S. units as judged by protective effect in the laboratory.

Animal sera are usually prepared in horses. On occasion, a different species may be used. In the past, cows, rabbits, and other animals were used for specific antibody stimulation. The reader is advised to consult the product brochure for any product containing animal sera to be certain of the species of origin and precautions in its use.

All animal sera have an intrinsic hazard if administered to individuals who are sensitive to any of its protein or other biologic constituents, or to any of the preservatives used to prolong its shelf-life. Commonly, phenol or an organic mercurial is included. Some patients sensitive to mercury may react to receipt of products preserved in this fashion. Horse antigen sensitivity can result in anaphylaxis or serum sickness. In an effort to eliminate or decrease this risk, a careful history followed by skin testing is essential.

The history must include inquiry about asthma, hay fever, urticaria, and other allergic reactions that followed either exposure to the animal in question or previous injections of serum from that species. Patients with a generalized history of asthma, vasomotor rhinitis, or other allergic symptoms may be sensitive, and great care should be exercised in administration of an animal serum product to these patients.

Sensitivity tests for serum reactions are best performed intracutaneously. Some allergists prefer a scratch or eye test prior to the intracutaneous route. The scratch test is performed by applying one drop of a 1 : 100 saline dilution of the serum onto the site of a superficial scratch and observing it within 15 to 30 minutes. A positive reaction consists of erythema or wheal formation.

The eye test is performed by instilling a drop of 1 : 10 saline dilution of serum in one eye and a drop of physiologic saline solution in the other eye to serve as a control. Positive reaction consists of lacrimation and conjunctivitis appearing in 10 to 30 minutes in the eye into which the serum dilution has been placed. Many allergists omit conjunctival testing in favor of scratch and intradermal tests.

If the scratch or eye test is negative, an intradermal test is performed by injecting 0.1 ml of a 1 : 100 saline dilution. This reaction is read after 10 to 30 minutes and is positive if a wheal appears. In persons with a history of allergy, the dose is reduced to 0.05 ml of a 1 : 1000 dilution intradermally. *Intradermal skin tests have resulted in fatalities. Scratch tests have not. Therefore, never inject a serum or perform a skin test unless a syringe containing 1 ml of 1 : 1000 aqueous epinephrine is within immediate reach and adequate personnel are available to administer it intravenously if necessary.*

Skin and eye tests indicate the probability of sensitivity. However, a negative skin or eye test is not an absolute guarantee of absence of sensitivity. With either a specific history of allergy or a positive skin or eye test, a decision must be made as to whether horse serum will be administered. If it is necessary to do so, the so-called desensitization procedure to be described would be used.

If the history and sensitivity tests are both negative, then the indicated dose of serum may be given intramuscularly. Intravenous injection may be indicated if it is important to achieve a high level of antibody immediately. In such instances, a preliminary dose of 0.5 ml of serum should be diluted in 10 ml of either physiologic saline or 5% glucose solution. This preparation should be given intravenously as slowly as possible and the patient watched for 30 minutes for a reaction. If no reaction occurs, the remainder of the serum, diluted 1 : 20, may be given at a rate not to exceed 1 ml/minute.

If it is necessary to desensitize an individual who has either a positive history or a positive screening test, then the following procedure should be used.

Make certain that epinephrine, 1 : 1000, is in a syringe and at hand. Serum is given slowly in order to tie up all of the preformed antibody present in the patient's serum. This results in establishing the tolerance level of the patient. The procedure is as follows: Every 15 minutes, inject the following, but only if there has been no reaction to the preceding dose:

1. 0.05 ml of a 1 : 20 dilution subcutaneously;
2. 0.1 ml of a 1 : 10 dilution subcutaneously;
3. 0.3 ml of a 1 : 10 dilution subcutaneously;
4. 0.1 ml undiluted serum subcutaneously;
5. 0.2 ml of undiluted serum subcutaneously;
6. 0.5 ml of undiluted serum intramuscularly.
7. Inject remaining therapeutic dose intramuscularly.

Serum reactions that have occurred following horse serum administration are of three types: (1) acute anaphylaxis; (2) serum sickness; and (3) acute febrile reactions.

Anaphylactic reactions are manifested by urticaria, dyspnea, cyanosis, shock, and occasionally unconsciousness. These reactions occur within seconds or minutes after an injection and must be considered critical emergencies.

Serum sickness reactions are delayed in onset and occur more frequently in persons who have previously received serum injections or who received large doses. These reactions consist of rash, urticaria, arthritis, adenopathy, and fever, occurring hours or days after the injection. If this is the reaction after a first exposure to serum, 7 to 12 days may elapse before the serum sickness syndrome occurs.

Febrile reactions after animal serum injections are usually mild because all licensed products have undergone pyrogenicity testing. Mild febrile reactions are usually of no significance. However, severe febrile reactions rarely result in death with hyperpyrexia as a major manifestation.

Treatment of serum reactions ranges from mild symptomatic therapy for mild serum sickness and mild fever to urgent therapy for anaphylactic reactions.

Aqueous epinephrine, 1 : 1000, is administered subcutaneously or intramuscularly immediately in a dose of 0.01 ml/kg body weight in anaphylactic reactions. If there is no immediate improvement, aqueous epinephrine, 1 : 1000, is administered intravenously at a dose of 0.01 ml/kg. For intravenous use, the 1 : 1000 concentration of epinephrine must be diluted to 1 : 10 in physiologic saline and injected slowly (maximum dose is 5 ml of this 1 : 10,000 resultant dilution). An intravenous infusion of physiologic saline should be begun immediately. Epinephrine may be repeated after 5 to 15 minutes if the response is not satisfactory. All other measures to sustain blood pressure and oxygenation should be employed as needed.

For severe urticaria or laryngeal edema, intramuscular injections of full doses of antihistamines are indicated in addition to epinephrine. Adrenal corticosteroids have little place in the treatment of acute reactions but may be employed with persistent and severe reactions. They should only be given after epinephrine and antihistamines have been administered and it has been determined that the reaction is persisting. Many experts advise administering 100 to 200 mg of hydrocortisone intravenously immediately and every 4 to 6 hours for as long as necessary. Alternatively, 40 to 80 mg of dexamethasone may be used. If serum therapy must be resumed, wait until all visible signs of reaction have subsided. This interval is often 6 to 8 hours in length.

On rare occasions, human plasma will be used in passive prophylaxis. This procedure is usually avoided in order to avert the risk of hepatitis virus transmission. With the availability of gamma globulin preparations, the use of human plasma to convey antibodies has been virtually eliminated. One area in which plasma continues to be useful is in patients deficient in B cells (antibodies) in whom gamma globulin has caused reaction. In such circumstances, plasma from a single, hepatitis-free donor is utilized (the so-called buddy system). It is beyond the scope of this text to detail its use in this circumstance. The reader is referred to immunology textbooks listed in the references for further reading.

REFERENCES

Bellanti J: Immunology II. Philadelphia, WB Saunders, 1979

Benacerraf B, Unanaue ER: Textbook of Immunology. Baltimore, Williams & Wilkins, 1979

Cooper MD, Dayton DH (eds): Development of Host Defenses. New York, Raven Press, 1977

Freedom SO, Gold P: Clinical Immunology, 2nd ed. Baltimore, Harper & Row, 1976

Fudenberg HA, Stites DP, Caldwell JL, Wells JV: Basic and Clinical Immunology, 2nd ed. Los Altos, Lange Medical Publishers, 1980

Krugman S, Katz S: Infectious Diseases of Children, 7th ed. St. Louis, C.V. Mosby, Co. 1981

Mudd S: Infectious Agents and Host Reactions. Philadelphia, WB Saunders, 1970

Pabst HF, Kreth HW: Ontogeny of the immune response as a basis of childhood disease. J Pediatr 97:519–534, 1980

Samter M: Immunologic Diseases, Vol 1, 3rd ed. Chicago, Little, Brown & Co, 1978

Stiehm ER, Fulginiti VA: Immunologic Disorders in Infants and Children, 2nd ed. Philadelphia, WB Saunders, 1980

3
Informed Consent in Immunization Practice

Vincent A. Fulginiti

This chapter will deal with an issue that has achieved prominence only in the past decade: the consent of an informed patient or of the patient's parent or guardian to a contemplated immunization. Strictly speaking, this is a legal, sociologic, and political topic. I am not a lawyer, sociologist, or politician. Hence, the discussion will not be cloaked with any of these authorities. Rather, I will attempt to give you a physician's viewpoint. My only credentials are a longtime concern with the issue and participation on several national panels attempting to resolve some facets of the problem.

Why include this topic at all? The reasons are both practical and timely. Informed consent is an issue in everyone's practice; it is a topic of national concern, of debate, and of irresolution. Those in practice and those just starting out are asking themselves just how far their responsibilities carry them. What is prudent? What is sensible? What is required?

I will explore some facets of this problem from the standpoint of immunization practice. For learned articles on the legal, sociologic, and political standpoints, the reader is referred to the list of appended references.

RESPONSIBILITIES AND RIGHTS OF THE
VARIOUS PARTIES IN IMMUNIZATION PRACTICE

I believe that the keynote of the informed consent issue is responsibility. All physicians wish to act in the best interest of their patients. What is in the best interest of the patient in terms of immunization? The answer is more complex than cursory examination suggests.

For the most part, an immunization encounter is a voluntary request by the patient for protection against future disease. *By "patient" I include here and hereafter parents and guardians acting on behalf of children who are patients.* The only current sociologic condition that tempers this voluntary relationship is the proliferation of school immunization laws that mandate complete vaccine receipt as a condition for entry and continuation in the classroom. Thus, some patients are seeking immunizations on a nonvoluntary basis.

Of course, some patients do not wish to be immunized. I will deal with this subject at a later point.

In the past, the voluntary request nature of immunization resulted in many physicians simply assuming that their judgment alone would suffice as to what vaccinations were needed and when. The statement, "It's time for your baby's shots," summarizes this viewpoint. Often the physician did little else in the way of explaining and simply proceeded to give whatever appeared appropriate. Society followed and approved this method, assuming that the professional standard of practice dictated such choices, and there was little litigation concerning immunization injury prior to the advent of live virus vaccines.

In my experience with teaching medical students and residents, I often quiz a parent *after* the well-baby encounter in order to illustrate the fact that the parent has little or no conception of what vaccines the child had received and only a vague appreciation of what the vaccines do in preventing disease. Many parents cannot name or list the diseases for which the immunizations were protective, simply referring to them as "baby shots" or a similar appellation. Furthermore, virtually none have any knowledge or idea of any adverse effects, other than fever and irritability, following diphtheria-tetanus-pertussis (DTP) vaccination.

I believe, as do others, that such observations have led to the question of physician responsibility. A physician's responsibility should be generated by concern in deciding what is in the patient's best interest. Although the simplistic answer is that we really don't know, many issues are involved in attempting to answer this question, and the following discussion summarizes these components.

Every member of our society has the right of individual choice. Such free choice occurs in various degrees. We can choose to get an education or not, to eat certain foods or not, and so on. In many other circumstances, our choices are limited only by what is available. Yet society sometimes imposes limits with penalties for exercising free choice; one cannot pass a red light without risking a fine.

Underlying this basic tenet of choice is the principle that (ideally) people will make good choices, and that they will do so because they are sufficiently knowledgeable of the benefits and risks of each choice.

We recognize that people do not always make sound choices, as exemplified by their smoking, drinking, speeding, and so on, and that they do not always know or may not consider benefits and risks. In medicine, it has been tacitly assumed by many that "choice" is not really in the patient's domain, but in the physician's. Can anyone conceive of a physician making a diagnosis of beta-hemolytic streptococcal pharyngitis and offering the patient a choice of no treatment versus penicillin? I cannot. The assumption in this type of encounter is that the physician knows best, *and this assumption is accepted by both patient and physician*, dictated by our common medical mores.

On the other hand, certain clinical situations have always been associated with some degree of choice. The most obvious example is when alternative forms of therapy, none of which is absolute, are contemplated for a disease in which the risks of the treatment are high and the benefits low. In most such clinical situations, the physician usually discusses the options and helps the patient to make a choice.

Between these extremes are all shades of choice and knowledge. Generalizations are of little use here, because the characteristics of patients and physicians, the specific clinical circumstances, and the degree of information given and received will determine the degree of choice afforded the patient. This vast area of medical practice is one of uncertainty, and it is here that much of immunization informed consent experience lies. There are many uncertainties that society has not resolved, and the practitioner is left with few or no guidelines for appropriate behavior.

In the past decade or so, the comfortable "physician-knows-best" method of medical functioning in immunization practice has been severely tested. Societal and legal forces have focused attention on the patient's right to know and to choose. Two major events in immunization practice have precipitated this concern more forcefully than other considerations. Also, the general litigious nature of medical encounters, with a multiplicity of malpractice suits, many ending successfully, have served as a background of anxiety and concern from which current practices are evolving.

Malpractice actions and the malpractice insurance crisis of the 1960s and 1970s alerted the public, the legal profession, legislators, and physicians to the general concept that medical negligence was a cause for legal redress. The first major immunization event occurred in 1974, when a child who had received live oral polio vaccine and had become paralyzed successfully sued for damages as a result of the intrinsic risk of the virus in the vaccine. Despite considerable scientific opinion to the contrary, the decision was upheld through all appellate courts and stands as a landmark in informed consent practice and the issue of liability.

The details of this case are important legally, but for our purposes need not be recited in detail. What are critical are the issues that arose afterwards suggesting that a patient about to receive vaccine should be informed of the risks and benefits and of any alternate choices.

The second immunization event was the now infamous swine influenza vaccine campaign of 1977. Some experts saw influenza as a major health hazard and urgent steps were taken to develop and administer influenza vaccine on a massive scale. What followed was the unexpected development of a complication, Guillain-Barre syndrome, with attendant morbidity and mortality. This entire effort and its consequences were front page news for weeks, and served to highlight the many informed consent issues for the public and for legislators.

All of this historical background is being provided to illustrate the uncertainties we now face as to just what is in the patient's best interest. If one looks at the issue solely from the standpoint of the individual, a forceful argument can be made that the patient has a right to know the following: (1) the risks of a given infectious disease if contracted; (2) the risk of an unimmunized person acquiring the disease; (3) the benefits to be derived from receiving a vaccine for that disease; and (4) the risks associated with receiving that vaccine.

Although such goals seem desirable, attaining them may prove totally impracticable. Can a lay person readily understand epidemiologic and statistical concepts involved in disease risk? Can a reasoned assessment be made of the value of a given vaccine? How does a lay person place a remote risk into a decision-making process? Some diehards argue that only a medical education would suffice to prepare someone for making such assessments.

Proponents of informed consent and individual rights argue that most people can grasp risk-benefits concepts and can choose wisely, if given the opportunity. Furthermore, they argue that the patient does, and should, have the right of refusal if the patient perceives the risk as greater than the benefits.

What, then, of the rights of society? If a person is allowed to decide whether or not he will receive a particular vaccine, does this mean that the rest of us must accept the possibility of disease in that person and of transmission to as yet unimmunized persons? Our society also has a tradition that in certain public health issues, the rights of all supercede the rights of any one person. For example, we do not permit salmonella carriers to handle food. In the past, smallpox vaccination was mandated under penalty of fine and even jail. Currently, in most jurisdictions, school attendance is denied to anyone not completely immunized.

This conflict between individual and group rights is still unresolved. Attempts to fuse the two viewpoints are found in disclaimer clauses in many school immunization laws that permit individual avoidance of their provisions. These are often made on religious grounds, but in many jurisdictions a patient need only express a desire not to be immunized. The final test in many areas is often legal action to determine which thread of law will prevail: that of the individual or that of the group.

In Arizona in 1980, the attorney general decided that schools could *not* exclude a student who had failed to receive mandated immunizations. In this state, the individual's rights appear paramount at present.

Does the physician enjoy any rights in this arena? What constitutes responsible action of a physician in recommending, prescribing, and administering vaccines? The answer is unclear. I believe that the physician must make a reasonable attempt to inform all patients of major benefits and risks, allow time for questions and discussion, and permit choice (more on this approach with specifics later).

Finally, there are the manufacturer's rights. In this country, we follow the common-law traditions of England with its tort provisions. As I understand this legal precept, a manufacturer must assure the quality of any product marketed. If a defective product is dispensed and a person is injured as a result, tort law provides that the injured party can seek legal redress. For more than 100 years, the concept of a contract between two parties has governed these relationships. For most products, the courts have been able to determine issues of liability, negligence, and the like. For pharmaceuticals, courts have been less certain of their grounds. One theme is that the court does not know what is safe and therefore can only determine safety after the fact. It is left to the experts to determine the safety margin of a given biologic product, and the court will consider issues of liability only if injury occurs and if action is taken against the manufacturer.

These traditions, along with burgeoning insurance, legal, and judgment costs have forced many manufacturers either to stop manufacturing vaccines or to seek methods by which they are "held harmless." The manufacturer of the swine influenza vaccine, for example, agreed to release the product only after the federal government had agreed to act as insurer and recipient of all claims of injury resulting from influenza vaccine administration.

This issue of intrinsic liability has potentially serious social consequences. For example, only a single drug company in the United States currently produces measles vaccine. Not only is competition stifled, but if the manufacturing process goes awry, all of us could be deprived of this important biologic product.

This brief, nonlegal, and unlearned discussion has been put forward to demonstrate the complexity of the issues involved in informed consent. I must again remind the reader that I am not a legal expert in this area.

THE NATURE OF INFORMED CONSENT

Leslie J. Miller from the Division of Corporate Law of the American Medical Association recently cited a court case in defining informed consent as, "The duty of the physician to explain the procedure to the patient and warn him of any material risks or damages inherent in, or collateral to, the therapy, so as to enable the patient to make an intelligent and informed choice about whether or not to undergo such treatment" (see *References*). This definition bears detailed examination in relation to immunization.

Informed consent has several discrete elements: (1) the implied duty of the physician; (2) the explanation to the patient; (3) the warning to the patient; (4) the enabling of intelligent choice by the patient; and (5) a yes or no decision.

Courts clearly see the provision of informed consent as the duty of the physician. The inescapable conclusion is that the physician *must* inform the patient. In many states, this duty is determined by the professional standard of practice in that community, and one does whatever is accepted as the usual practice in one's legal geographic area. In Arizona, for example, this is the standard against which an individual physician's actions are judged.

In some parts of the country, and in more recent times, the duty of the physician has been defined by the patient's need to know and not by what other physicians do. Legally, this is referred to as the material risk approach and under it, the concept of a universal standard in a given area is rejected in favor of the degree of risk the patient faces with a given choice of action. The physician must responsibly recognize what the patient needs to know to make the choice.

"Explanation to the patient" encompasses the area most difficult to define. There is more uncertainty in this area than in any other part of informed consent, and fewer guidelines are available. What should be explained? What degree of comprehension should the patient be expected to attain? Does the responsibility of explanation lie with the physician or can it be delegated? Is a written explanation satisfactory? Often these issues are decided in the individual case with heavy reliance on expert testimony and textbook and literature citation to establish how much information is enough. Also influencing this consideration are the other facets of the definition.

Has the patient been warned of inherent risks and dangers of immunization? Does one need to disclose information about a serious but very rare complication of vaccine administration? For example, should the patient be informed that encephalitis may follow live measles virus vaccine, even though it is uncertain whether it is causally related to the vaccine virus, and is extremely rare? It again appears that it is the individual circumstances, coupled with expert testimony, that determine which "truth" is believed in a court of law. This makes it difficult to anticipate, in advance of action taken, just what the answers to these questions should be.

Finally, if injury actually occurs, it must be evident that disclosure of risk could have enabled the patient to avoid the adverse consequence. This implies that the patient had been given sufficient information to choose, with "no" as a possible response. The unembellished statement, "It's time for your baby's shots," falls far short of all aspects of the definition of informed consent.

THE USE OF FORMS

In an effort to document many medical procedures involving informed consent, specific forms have been developed with written provision of information needed by the patient. Usually such forms contain provision for a patient's signature to indicate consent. In many instances, the use of such forms is the focus for a relaxed discussion between the doctor and the patient, an opportunity for questions and reflection, and ultimate consent indicating comprehension and the patient's willingness to accept the procedure. In other instances, the form has become shorthand for routine; the patient is told what will happen and signature is requested without any discussion, questions, or reflection.

An informed-consent document is only as good as the procedure with which it is used. If the physician supplies the patient with a legible form listing in lay language the principal benefits and risks of a given immunization, and then permits time for explanation and questions, the form has served a useful purpose. If it is shoved under the patient's nose with a request to sign it, the form might just as well never have existed.

Immunization forms currently available from the Center for Disease Control (CDC) will be discussed shortly, but before this, some aspects of the use of forms should be considered.

First, any form should be specific. General forms simply do not provide enough detail to enable the patient to make an intelligent choice. If the physician is about to administer poliovirus vaccine, the form must be specific to that disease and that vaccine.

Second, the form must be in clear language, understandable to a nonmedical person. "Brain fever" is a better term than "encephalitis." But whatever the language used, the physician should always ask the patient if all the terms are understood.

Third, the form should contain benefit and risk information for both the disease to be prevented and the vaccine to be used.

Fourth, if there is a choice among different types of vaccines, details for each should be provided with separate risk-benefit statements.

Use of the form must include opportunity for questions, for explanation and discussion, and for final decision making by the patient. Generally, a signature of the responsible person is obtained and should be witnessed by a third party. The physician should then include in his note of the encounter that the form was presented, read, and discussed.

FACTORS IN INFORMED CONSENT FOR RECEIPT OF IMMUNIZATIONS

THE KNOWLEDGE OF PHYSICIANS

Anyone who administers vaccines should be aware of the benefits and risks of any product used. All discussion of informed consent is worthless if the physician himself is uninformed. One cannot expect the blind to lead the blind in medical practice. Of course, I am referring to risks that are known and documented and about which information is readily available. In many circumstances in immunization practice, risks cannot be anticipated prior to widespread use of the vaccine.

The sources for vaccine information are legion, with varying degrees of authority and completeness. Two major national advisory bodies — the American Academy of Pediatrics (AAP) and the CDC — issue periodic vaccine and other biologic product recommendations.

The AAP maintains a standing committee on infectious disease (the Redbook Committee). Approximately every three to four years, a comprehensive manual of infectious diseases is published which contains discussions of the major diseases and vaccines, and recommendations for preventive measures. This manual, commonly known as the *Redbook*, is supplemented by committee statements on specific issues, which are periodically published between the dates of release of the *Redbook*. These are published in the journal *Pediatrics* and are disseminated to all members of the AAP. All such recommendations are considered opinions of a group of experts that reflect their best judgment at the time. Their recommendations are often based on solid data and undergo very little change over time. Data on some issues are incomplete or unavailable but practice needs demand some guidelines. The committee seeks to resolve such issues of uncertainty by outlining the available data and making reasonable recommendations. Not every expert agrees with every such recommendation.

The CDC maintains a standing committee, the Advisory Committee on Immunization Practices (ACIP). This group makes its recommendations in *Morbidity and Mortality Weekly Report* (MMWR), a weekly publication available to any physician for the asking. Drop a postcard to the CDC in Atlanta, Georgia, and your name will be added to the mailing list.

In addition to these two sources, a third compilation is periodically published by the American Public Health Association. This is entitled *Control of Communicable Diseases in Man* and takes a much more global viewpoint, detailing both vaccine information and considerable data on etiology, epidemiology, and other measures in the control of communicable diseases.

In addition to these standard recognized sources, there are other, less frequently consulted publications, such as *Health Information for International Travel*, a very useful pamphlet published annually by the CDC which serves as a guide to the specific immunization requirements of various countries. It can be obtained from the Superintendant of Documents, U.S. Government Printing Office, Washington, D.C. 20402. It is routinely sent to all subscribers to MMWR.

Pediatric and other journals are another source of information. Original and review articles concerning immunization are often published in *Pediatrics, The Journal of Pediatrics, The American Journal of Diseases of Children, Clinical Pediatrics, The Journal of the American Medical Association, The New England Journal of Medicine,* and *The Journal of Infectious Diseases.* In addition, *The American Journal of Public Health* and *Public Health Reports* often contain articles on immunization that are of interest to practitioners.

Another source of vaccine information is selected reading in pediatric and other texts. Unfortunately, most standard texts offer little comprehensive or complete commentary on immunization. Among textbooks suggested as partial guides to authoritative sources of information are those listed in the references at the end of this chapter.

Experts at various medical schools throughout the country, in local and state public health departments, and at the CDC can be consulted for specific information. Letters and phone calls are accepted and prompt response is the rule.

Finally, public health agencies in most cities, counties, and states have individuals active in immunization practice. Up-to-date information about epidemiology of disease and immunization requirements and recommendations can be provided. These agencies are also particularly adept at providing information about nursery school, school, public health, and foreign travel concerns, as well as other matters relating to public health issues.

THE STANDARD OF PRACTICE

National advisory bodies present recommendations for general use but they cannot anticipate all local circumstances or all problems that are likely to arise in administration of vaccines. For example, the indications for rabies prophylaxis will vary considerably throughout the United States, depending on the species of animals infected in the area. What is standard in Arizona may represent bad practice in Montana in any given year.

Thus, local and state health departments can be invaluable sources of disease data which might alter use of some biologics, deviating from otherwise acceptable recommendations. Further, legal requirements differ from state to state, and local statutes often determine the nature and extent of informed consent procedures.

A physician is ill advised to employ immunization practices that deviate markedly from local circumstances. Thus, if every individual practitioner in an area obtains some form of informed consent in writing, it would be foolish for a physician to not incorporate such a standard into his practice. As was mentioned, many legal jurisdictions depend heavily on the professional standard of practice as the guideline for a specific incident. This consideration alone often mandates the way in which informed consent is obtained and recorded.

EMERGENCIES

Most immunization practice is elective but in an emergency, one may need to provide a vaccine or antibody preparation to a patient who is unresponsive and therefore cannot give consent. Tetanus immunization or immune globulin may be necessary in a severely traumatized unconscious patient. The usual procedures that apply to emergencies should be followed, including an attempt to contact and obtain consent from responsible relatives of the patient. However, in some circumstances, even this will not be possible, and the procedure must be performed. In such cases, the overriding concerns are whether the procedure is mandated by sound medical practice and whether the patient would be injured if the procedure were not followed.

THE QUESTION OF DELEGATION OF RESPONSIBILITY

Although it is common practice to delegate the administration of vaccines to ancillary health care personnel, the informed consent procedure should be carried out by a physician. Again, this issue is usually considered only in retrospect but if a physician has not discussed vaccine benefits and risk and an injury results, this fact may be held against him. The issues here seem more completely resolved in areas other than immunization practice. For example, consent to surgery should be obtained by the person who is to perform the surgery rather than by a ward nurse or even by another physician. It is less clear whether immunization informed consent can be delegated to another party. Even if it is delegated, the physician still retains ultimate responsibility for all aspects of the informed consent process.

THE QUESTION OF RECORDS

In many malpractice or negligence suits, the physician is particularly at risk if there is inadequate documentation of what was done and how it was done. Every report of an immunization procedure should include an indication that informed consent was given, specifics about the vaccine used, and indications of advice about untoward effects. It is particularly important to include the manufacturer, the lot number, and the expiration date of the vaccine in the patient's record at the time of immunization. This routine should become ingrained in office practice. Sometimes an individual lot of vaccine will have a particular complication associated with it. By following this routine, it will be relatively easy to determine which patients received the product and to undertake responsible surveillance for complications. Conversely, if there is an untoward reaction not attributable to a specific vaccine, such documentation may again be very useful. For example, if a patient experiences mercury hypersensitivity and attempts to attribute it to the vaccine or biologic used, it obviously would be useful to indicate that the actual vaccine or biologic used did not contain a mercurial preservative.

SOME GENERAL CONSIDERATIONS

The physician is well advised not to undertake immunization procedures unusual to his practice without first obtaining adequate information and consultation. For example, a pediatrician might be tempted to immunize the parent of one of his patients upon request. If the parent has complicated underlying disease, which may or may not be discernible by the pediatrician, an untoward and unanticipated result may occur.

In general, one should not guarantee results that are not 100% predictable, and a physician in immunization practice should always indicate that no vaccine is 100% protective. Thus, someone who has received live measles vaccine at an appropriate age under appropriate circumstances and still gets measles should have been alerted to this possibility by the physician. In fact, 3% to 5% of all those who receive live measles virus vaccine might not be protected, and this fact should have been made known to the patient, both in writing and in discussion.

The physician should ensure that adequate follow-up procedures are indicated to the patient once an immunization is undertaken. For example, if DTP is given to an infant, adequate care should be provided in the event of a severe febrile reaction. At the onset of the procedure, the physician should have indicated what procedures the patient should follow should such an adverse effect occur. This is not unique to immunization practice but it is particularly pertinent when certain reactions can be anticipated following vaccine administration.

One should always be certain that everyone in the office or clinic who is working with immunizations understands as clearly as the physician does each of the items discussed in this chapter. It is important that consistency be maintained in what the patient is told and in what is recorded.

A PRAGMATIC APPROACH TO INFORMED CONSENT IN IMMUNIZATION PRACTICE

The following steps are recommended towards ensuring that adequate informed consent communication has occurred:

1. Use some form of printed statement about the benefits and risks of the specific disease and vaccine. I am including in this chapter samples of documents, *Important Information About. . .* (see pp. 41–44). These documents have been prepared by the CDC for the major routine immunizations used in children. They are not perfect and are not issued by the CDC with any sort of mandate for their use in private practice. However, they are used extensively in the public health sector and by many practitioners and clinics. Their virtue is that a considered statement is made about the benefits and risks of both a specific disease and its vaccine. It is assumed that an intelligent person reading such statements would conclude that the vaccine is beneficial and should be received. It is also assumed that information about risks is sufficient to enable the patient to make an informed and intelligent decision.

Some physicians prefer to use forms of their own; in these instances, the CDC forms can serve as models for comparison. Whatever form is used, it should follow the characteristics indicated in this chapter.

2. At each and every immunization encounter, assign a short period of time for physician-patient contact. During this time ask the patient if the document about that immunization has been read and understood. Solicit questions and offer explanations if necessary. And, finally, obtain the

(Text continues on P. 45.)

ARIZONA DEPARTMENT OF HEALTH SERVICES

IMPORTANT INFORMATION ABOUT MEASLES, MUMPS AND RUBELLA AND MEASLES, MUMPS AND RUBELLA VACCINES

Please read this carefully

WHAT IS MEASLES? Measles is the most serious of the common childhood diseases. Usually it causes a rash, high fever, cough, runny nose, and watery eyes lasting 1 to 2 weeks. Sometimes it is more serious. It causes an ear infection or pneumonia in nearly 1 out of 10 children who get it. One child out of every 1,000 who get measles has an inflammation of the brain (encephalitis). This can lead to convulsions, deafness, or mental retardation. One child in every 10,000 who get measles dies from it. Measles can also cause a pregnant woman to have a miscarriage or possibly a deformed baby.

Before measles vaccine shots were available there were hundreds of thousands of cases each year. Nearly all children got measles by the time they were 15. Now, because of the wide use of measles vaccine, a child's risk of getting measles is much lower. However, if children stop getting vaccinated, the risk of getting measles will go right back up again.

WHAT IS MUMPS? Mumps is a common disease of children. Usually it causes fever, headache, and inflammation of the salivary glands, which causes the cheeks to swell. Sometimes it is more serious. It causes a mild type of meningitis in about 1 child in every 20 who get it. More rarely, it can cause inflammation of the brain (encephalitis) which usually goes away without leaving permanent damage. Mumps can also cause deafness. About 1 out of every 4 adult men who get mumps develops painful inflammation and swelling of the testicles. This usually goes away and rarely makes them sterile.

Before mumps vaccine shots were available, there were more than 150,000 cases each year. Now, because of the increasing use of mumps vaccine, the risk of getting mumps is much lower. However, if children stop getting vaccinated, the risk of getting mumps will go right back up again.

WHAT IS RUBELLA? Rubella is also called German measles. It is a common disease of children and may also affect adults. Usually it is very mild and causes a slight fever, rash, and swelling of glands in the neck. The sickness lasts about 3 days. Sometimes, especially in adult women, there may be swelling and aching of the joints for a week or two. Very rarely, rubella can cause inflammation of the brain (encephalitis) or cause abnormal bleeding.

If a pregnant woman gets rubella, there's a good chance that she may have a miscarriage or that the child will be born crippled, blind, or with other defects. The last big rubella epidemic in the United States was in 1964. After it was over, about 25,000 children were born with serious problems such as deformities,

heart problems, deafness, blindness, or mental retardation because their mothers had rubella during the pregnancy.

Before rubella vaccine shots were available, rubella was so common that most children got it by the time they were 15. Now, because of the wide use of rubella vaccine, the risk of getting rubella is much lower. However, if children stop getting vaccinated, the risk of getting rubella or having a defective baby because of rubella infection during pregnancy will go right back up again.

MEASLES, MUMPS, AND RUBELLA VACCINES: Immunization is one of the best ways to prevent these diseases. The vaccines are given by injection and are very effective. In about 90% of people, one shot will give protection, probably for life. Since protection may not be quite as good if the vaccines are given very early in life, these vaccines should be given to children after their first birthday; measles vaccine should be given at 15 months of age or older. Measles, mumps, and rubella vaccines can be given as individual injections or in a combined form by a single injection. If they are given in combined form, they should be given at 15 months of age or older.

Experts recommend that women of childbearing age who are not known to be immune to rubella should receive the vaccine if they are not pregnant and will not become pregnant for 3 months. Adolescent and adult males who do not have a history of vaccination or a blood test showing that they are immune should be vaccinated.

POSSIBLE SIDE EFFECTS FROM THE VACCINES: About 1 out of every 5 children will get a rash or slight fever 1 or 2 weeks after getting measles vaccine. Occasionally there is a mild swelling of the salivary glands after mumps vaccination. Although experts are not sure, it seems that very rarely children who get these vaccines may have a more serious reaction, such as inflammation of the brain (encephalitis), convulsions with fever, or nerve deafness.

About 1 out of every 7 children who get rubella vaccine will get a rash or some swelling of the glands of the neck 1 or 2 weeks after the shot. About 1 out of every 20 children who get rubella vaccine will have some aching or swelling of the joints. This may happen anywhere from 2 to 10 weeks after the shot. It usually lasts only 2 or 3 days. Adults are more likely to have these problems with their joints—as many as 1 in 4 may have them. Other side effects, such as pain, numbness, or tingling in the hands and feet have also occurred but are very uncommon.

With any vaccine or drug, there is a possibility that allergic or other more serious reactions or even death could occur.

WARNING—SOME PERSONS SHOULD *NOT* TAKE THESE VACCINES WITHOUT CHECKING WITH A DOCTOR:

- Those who are sick right now with something more serious than a cold.
- Those with allergy to an antibiotic called neomycin.
- Those with cancer or leukemia or lymphoma.
- Those with diseases that lower the body's resistance to disease.
- Those taking drugs that lower the body's resistance to infection, such as cortisone or prednisone.
- Those who have received gamma globulin within the preceding 3 months.

PREGNANCY: Vaccine experts do not know if measles or mumps vaccines can cause special problems for pregnant women or their unborn babies. However, doctors usually avoid giving any drugs or vaccines to pregnant women unless there is a specific need. To be safe, pregnant women should not routinely get measles or mumps vaccine. A woman who gets measles or mumps vaccines should wait 3 months before getting pregnant.

Because rubella disease can cause severe problems for pregnant women or their unborn babies, it is possible that rubella vaccine might also cause these problems. Pregnant women should not get rubella shots. A woman who gets a rubella shot should wait 3 months before getting pregnant.

Vaccinating a child whose mother is pregnant is not dangerous to the pregnancy.

QUESTIONS: If you have any questions about measles, mumps or rubella vaccination, please ask us now or call your doctor or health department before you sign this form.

REACTIONS: If the person who received the vaccine gets sick and visits a doctor, hospital, or clinic in the 4 weeks after vaccination, please report it to your county health department.

I have read the information on this form about MEASLES, MUMPS AND RUBELLA AND MEASLES, MUMPS AND RUBELLA VACCINES. I have had a chance to ask questions which were answered to my satisfaction. I believe I understand the benefits and risks of measles vaccines and request that the vaccine checked below by given to me or to the person named below for whom I am authorized to make this request. This form and any information thereon may be transmitted to the State and County Health Departments for the purpose of administering the immunization program.

VACCINE TO BE GIVEN:

☐ MEASLES ☐ MUMPS ☐ RUBELLA
☐ MEASLES/RUBELLA ☐ MEASLES/MUMPS/RUBELLA

INFORMATION ON PERSON TO RECEIVE VACCINE

NAME (Please Print)		BIRTHDATE	AGE
ADDRESS			
CITY	COUNTY		
STATE		ZIPCODE	
SIGNATURE OF PARENT, GUARDIAN OR PERSON AUTHORIZED TO MAKE THE REQUEST			DATE

FOR CLINIC USE

SCHOOL OR CLINIC IDENTIFICATION	
VACCINE GIVEN	DATE VACCINATED
MANUFACTURER AND LOT NO	SITE OF INJECTION

ADHS/DCS/Disease Prevention and Epidemiology-114 (Rev. 4-81)

IMPORTANT INFORMATION ABOUT DIPHTHERIA, TETANUS AND PERTUSSIS AND DTP AND Td VACCINES

Please read this carefully

WHAT IS DIPHTHERIA? Diphtheria is a very serious disease which can affect people in different ways. It can cause an infection in the nose and throat which can interfere with breathing. It can also cause an infection of the skin. Sometimes it causes heart failure and paralysis. About 1 person out of every 10 who get diphtheria dies of it.

WHAT IS TETANUS? Tetanus, or lockjaw, results when wounds are infected with tetanus bacteria, which often live in dirt. The bacteria in the wound make a poison which causes the muscles of the body to go into spasm. Six out of every 10 persons who get tetanus die of it.

WHAT IS PERTUSSIS? Pertussis, or whooping cough, causes severe spells of coughing which can interfere with breathing. It also often causes pneumonia. Convulsions, brain damage, and death may occur, most often in very young infants.

Before vaccines were developed, these 3 diseases were all very common and caused a large number of deaths each year in the United States. Even now, hundreds of cases occur each year. If children stop getting vaccinated, the number of cases will go up again.

DTP and Td VACCINES: Immunization with DTP vaccine is one of the best ways to prevent these diseases. DTP vaccine is actually 3 vaccines combined into 1 to make it easier to get protection. The vaccine is given by injection starting early in infancy. Several doses are needed to get good protection. Young children should get 3 doses in the first year of life and a fourth dose at about 18 months of age. A booster dose is important for children and should be given between the ages of 4 and 6.

The vaccine is very effective at preventing tetanus—over 95% of those who get the vaccine are protected if the recommended number of shots is given. Although the diphtheria and pertussis parts of the vaccine are not quite as effective, they still prevent most children from getting the disease and they make the disease milder for those who do get it. Because pertussis is not very common in older children and because reactions to the pertussis part of the vaccine may be more common in older children, those 7 years of age and older should take a form of the vaccine that does not contain the pertussis part. This is called Td vaccine. Boosters with the Td vaccine should be gotten every 10 years throughout life.

POSSIBLE SIDE EFFECTS FROM THE VACCINES: Most children will have a slight fever and be irritable sometime in the day or 2 after taking the shot. Sometimes children develop some soreness and swelling in the area where the shot was given. About 1 out of every 7,000 children who get the shots will have a more serious side effect such as: high fever, convulsions, abnormal crying for several hours, or going into shock and getting pale. Rarely, about once in every 100,000 shots, inflammation of the brain (encephalitis) or brain damage may occur. Death may occur, even more rarely.

WARNING—SOME PERSONS SHOULD *NOT* TAKE THESE VACCINES WITHOUT CHECKING WITH A DOCTOR:

- Those who are sick right now with something more serious than a cold.
- Those who have had convulsions or other problems of the nervous system.
- Those who have had serious reactions to DTP shots before.

QUESTIONS: If you have any questions about diphtheria, tetanus, or pertussis or DTP vaccination, please ask us now or call your doctor or health department before you sign this form.

REACTIONS: If the person who received the vaccine gets sick and visits a doctor, hospital or clinic in the 4 weeks after vaccination, please report it to your county health department.

I have read the information on this form about DIPHTHERIA, TETANUS, AND PERTUSSIS AND DTP, and Td VACCINES. I have had a chance to ask questions which were answered to my satisfaction. I believe I understand the benefits and risks of DTP and Td vaccines and request that it be given to me or to the person named below for whom I am authorized to make this request. This form and any information thereon may be transmitted to the State and County Health Departments for the purpose of administering the immunization program.

INFORMATION ON PERSON TO RECEIVE VACCINE

NAME (Please Print)		BIRTHDATE	AGE
ADDRESS			
CITY	COUNTY		
STATE		ZIPCODE	
SIGNATURE OF PARENT, GUARDIAN OR PERSON AUTHORIZED TO MAKE THE REQUEST			DATE

FOR CLINIC USE

SCHOOL OR CLINIC IDENTIFICATION	DATE VACCINATED
MANUFACTURER AND LOT NO.	SITE OF INJECTION

ADHS/DCS/Disease Prevention and Epidemiology-101 (Rev. 4-81)

ARIZONA DEPARTMENT OF HEALTH SERVICES

IMPORTANT INFORMATION ABOUT POLIO AND POLIO VACCINE

Please read this carefully

WHAT IS POLIO? Polio is a virus disease that often causes permanent crippling (paralysis). One person out of every 10 who get polio disease dies from it. There used to be thousands of cases and hundreds of deaths from polio every year in the United States. Since polio vaccine became available in the mid-1950's, polio has nearly been eliminated. In the last five years, fewer than 25 cases have been reported each year. It's hard to say exactly what the risk is of getting polio at the present. Even for someone who is not vaccinated, the risk is very low. However, if we do not keep our children protected by vaccination the risk of polio will go back up again.

ORAL LIVE POLIO VACCINE: Immunization with oral live polio vaccine is one of the best ways to prevent polio. It is given by mouth starting in early infancy. Several doses are needed to provide good protection. Young children should get two doses in the first year of life and another dose at about 18 months of age. A booster dose is important for children when they enter school or when there is a high risk of polio, for example during an epidemic or when traveling to a place where polio is common. The vaccine is easy to take, effective in preventing the spread of polio, and, in over 90% of people, gives protection for a long time, probably for life.

POSSIBLE SIDE EFFECTS FROM THE VACCINE: Oral live polio vaccine rarely produces side effects. However, once in about every 4 million vaccinations, persons who have been vaccinated or who come in close contact with those who have recently been vaccinated are permanently crippled and may die. Even though these risks are very low, they should be recognized. The risk of side effects from the vaccine must be balanced against the risk of the disease, both now and in the future.

PREGNANCY: Polio vaccine experts do not think oral polio vaccine can cause special problems for pregnant women or their unborn babies. However, doctors usually avoid giving any drugs or vaccines to pregnant women unless there is a specific need. Pregnant women should check with a doctor before taking oral polio vaccine.

WARNING—SOME PERSONS SHOULD *NOT* TAKE ORAL POLIO VACCINE WITHOUT CHECKING WITH A DOCTOR:

- Those with cancer or leukemia or lymphoma.
- Those with diseases that lower the body's resistance to infection.
- Those taking drugs that lower the body's resistance to infection, such as cortisone or prednisone.
- Those who live in the same household with any of the above persons.
- Those who are sick right now with something more serious than a cold.
- Pregnant women.
- Most persons over the age of 18 because adults have a slightly bigger risk of developing paralysis from oral polio vaccine than children. (However, if the risk of polio is increased—as may occur, for example, when there is an outbreak in your community—polio experts recommend that unprotected persons receive oral polio vaccine regardless of age.

NOTE ON INJECTABLE (KILLED) POLIO VACCINE: Besides the oral polio vaccine, there is also a killed polio vaccine given by injection which protects against polio after several shots. It has no known risk of causing paralysis. Many polio experts feel that oral vaccine is more effective for controlling polio in the United States. Injectable polio vaccine is recommended for persons needing polio vaccination who have low resistance to infections or who live with persons with low resistance to infections. It may also be recommended for unprotected adults who plan to travel to a place where polio is common. It is not widely used in this country at the present time, but it is available. If you would like to know more about this type of polio vaccine, please ask us.

QUESTIONS: If you have any questions abut polio or polio vaccination, please ask us now or call your doctor or health department before you sign this form.

REACTIONS: If the person who received the vaccine gets sick and visits a doctor, hospital, or clinic in the 4 weeks after vaccination, please report it to your County Health Department.

ADHS/OCS/Epidemiology and Disease Prevention/EDP-102 (Rev. 7-80)

I have read the information on this form about POLIO AND THE ORAL VACCINE. I have had a chance to ask questions which were answered to my satisfaction. I believe I understand the benefits and risks of oral polio vaccine and request that it be given to me or to the person named below for whom I am authorized to make this request. This form and any information thereon may be transmitted to the State and County Health Departments for the purpose of administering the immunization program.

INFORMATION ON PERSON TO RECEIVE VACCINE

NAME (Please Print) | BIRTHDATE | AGE

ADDRESS

CITY | COUNTY

STATE | ZIPCODE

SIGNATURE OF PERSON TO RECEIVE VACCINE OR PERSON AUTHORIZED TO MAKE THE REQUEST | DATE

FOR CLINIC USE

SCHOOL OR CLINIC IDENTIFICATION

DATE VACCINATED

MANUFACTURER AND LOT NO.

ROUTE OF ADMINISTRATION OR SITE OF INJECTION

patient's written request for the immunization to be administered. Experts are divided as to the value of a signature; all consider that documentation in the physician's record is a more critical component.

3. Make an entry into the patient's permanent record that includes the signed consent form plus a note indicating that the encounter has occurred. In addition, the record should clearly state which vaccine was used and its manufacturer, its lot number, and its expiration date. The timing and nature of any reaction to the vaccine and any diagnostic or therapeutic measures that were undertaken should also be carefully recorded.

4. Make sure the patient has a clear indication of what procedures should be followed in the event of an adverse reaction to the vaccine.

5. At the next clinical encounter, ask whether the patient experienced any effects following the vaccination. Record any effects, or the absence of effects.

6. Should there be any adverse reactions that are significant or that differ from those previously reported for the vaccine, notify the manufacturer and the local health department. In the lattter case, it is anticipated that the information will be transmitted to the CDC's Division of Immunization.

If these procedures are followed and the usual doctor-patient relationship is maintained, few legal difficulties should be encountered. In the unfortunate event that such difficulties do occur, the physician will have accurate documentation of good medical practice to back him up.

THE FUTURE OF INFORMED CONSENT

It is impossible to predict whether universal standards will be adopted or mandated at the federal, regional, or state level. The uncertainties inherent in the tort process coupled with the uncertainties detailed in this chapter have led me to believe that it will be very difficult to precisely define all possible actions the physician should take. In some states, attempts are being made to codify the information necessary for certain procedures such as operations. These attempts include definition of just what the patient should be told from among the very many possible complications attendant on any one procedure. The results are very sketchy and fewer than a dozen procedures have been outlined in this fashion. In immunization practice, the CDC documents come the closest to an attempt at codification. However, the CDC is careful to disclaim any such authority for the documents, because at present they have no legal status. Such codification may become imperative, however, depending on what transpires concerning vaccine liability compensation. Some form of universal vaccine compensation is the most likely solution to the problem of informed consent in immunization practice. Several preliminary attempts in this direction have been made in the U.S. Some years ago, the Department of Health, Education, and Welfare studied the problem internally and asked a consulting company to estimate the scope of risk following administration of common vaccines, and the cost that would be incurred from compensation of injury. The assumption here is that vaccines have intrinsic risks, since they are biologic agents, and that even with careful, proper manufacturing procedures, such risks cannot be eliminated. For example, current oral polio vaccine is a live virus that on rare occasions causes paralysis. This is not related to negligence in manufacturing or administration; it is an intrinsic property of polio virus. A further assumption is that if the public health is to be served, some individuals may experience the intrinsic adverse side-effects of the vaccines used.

Combining these two assumptions, many have felt that the liability should be spread over the entire population benefiting from the immunization. Two avenues have been actively pursued. The first is for the manufacturers to slightly increase the cost of each vaccine and thus develop a vaccine compensation fund. The second is for the federal government to assume this responsibility out of tax generated funds. At present, neither approach has found favor, nor has any vaccine compensation plan been developed to the point that its use seems imminent.

There are several reasons why there is no vaccine compensation fund. First, the extent of liability appears to be enormous, conceivably amounting to billions of dollars, depending on the extent of and the value placed upon each of the possible adverse effects. Second, there is no universally accepted system for deciding whether a vaccine complication has occurred. Third, the tradition of individual capability to take action under the tort system is an extremely strong one in the United States. Some argue that even with a vaccine compensation plan, the individual has the right to pursue the matter through the court system.

Thus, it is unclear exactly how the current trends in informed consent will evolve. Most likely, some kind of uniform statutory regulation concerning the procedure to be followed will be developed at either the state or national level. Less likely in the immediate future, but under active consideration, is the possibility of a vaccine compensation plan that would obviate the need for legal intervention.

REFERENCES

American Surgical Association: Statement on professional liability, September 1976. New Engl J Med 295:1292–1296, 1976

Baynes TE, Jr: Liability for vaccine-related injuries: Public health considerations and some reflections on the swine flu experience. Leg Med Ann 1978:195–224

Bernzweig EP: The need for a national policy on injury reparations. New Engl J Med 296:569–571, 1977

Curran WJ: Drug company liability in immunization programs. New Engl J Med 281:1057–1058, 1969

Dandoy S: Communicable disease legislation. Ariz Med 23:735–736, 1976

Dowdle WR, Millar JD: Swine influenza: Lessons learned. Med Clin North Am 62:1047–1057, 1978

Editorial. Vaccination and the state. Lancet 1:605–666, 1974

Farber ME, Finkelstein SM: A cost-benefit analysis of a mandatory premarital rubella-antibody screening program. New Engl J Med 300:856–859, 1979

Hennessen W, Huygelen, C (eds): Immunization: Benefits versus risk factors (symposium). Develop Biol Stand 43:i–xii, 1–476, 1979

Krugman RD: Immunization "dyspractice." The need for "no fault" insurance. Pediatrics 56:159–160, 1975

Ladimer I: Mass immunizations: Legal problems and a proposed solution. J Commun Health 2:189–208, 1977

Melnick JL: Viral vaccines: New problems and prospects. Hosp Pract 13:104–112, 1978

Miller LJ: Informed consent: I. JAMA 244:2100–2103, 1980

Miller LJ: Informed consent: II. JAMA 244:2347–2351, 1980

Miller LJ: Informed consent: III. JAMA 244:2556–2558, 1980

Miller LJ: Informed consent: IV. JAMA 244:2661–2662, 1980

Rhomberg MA: OTA study assesses federal vaccine-related policies and options. Am J Hosp Pharm 37:135–137, 1980

Schumacher W: Legal/ethical aspects of vaccinations. Develop Biol Stand 43:435–438, 1979

Tondel LM: A lawyer looks at the "medical malpractice crisis". New Engl J Med 295:1315–1317, 1976

4

Practical Aspects of Immunization Practice

Vincent A. Fulginiti

Any physician who performs immunization procedures needs to establish personnel and office or clinic procedures which ensure safe and effective delivery of the vaccines. This chapter deals with the practical aspects of administering vaccines, from receipt and storage of vaccine products through individual administration practices to accurate recording of immunization data.

ESTABLISHING AN IMMUNIZATION STATION

In most offices and clinics, where the vast majority of vaccines are administered, adequate provision must be made for equipment, medications, and space. Many practitioners have established a separate area for administering immunizations, and the patient is referred to this area after being examined by the physician or health care personnel. Alternatively, immunizations may be administered at the same site where the primary medical encounter has occurred. The former method has the advantage of routinization of immunization procedures and equipment and the latter the disadvantage of necessitating mobility of vaccines and equipment into numerous areas.

Whichever site is chosen for administering vaccines, the area should contain adequate storage for the multiplicity of biologic products. Both a freezer and a refrigerator of adequate size should be readily available.

The refrigerator and freezer compartments should conform to temperature specifications because many biologic products are inactivated if the ambient temperature is not maintained. The following guidelines have been suggested in order to ensure stability of vaccines.*

Never store vaccines in areas of the refrigerator that are subject to wide temperature variations such as the shelves on the door. Instead, store them in areas such as the internal compartments where the temperature is more constant. When transporting vaccines from the place of purchase to the office or clinic, use styrofoam containers with ice packs for vaccines that need to be refrigerated and dry ice for vaccines that need to be kept frozen.

Keep polio vaccine in the frozen state at 14°F or lower. Ordinarily, polio vaccine will have a 12-month expiration date when maintained under these conditions. Live virus vaccines for measles, rubella, and mumps are extremely sensitive to exposure to light and warming. The live virus in these vaccines will be destroyed by exposure to ultraviolet light either before or after reconstitution; store these vaccines in the refrigerator at temperatures between 35.6°F and 46.4°F and protect them from light.

Store all products containing various combinations of diphtheria, pertussis, or tetanus antigens at temperatures ranging from 35°F to 46°F and *do not freeze them.*

Reconstituted vaccines vary in their stability. Unopened poliomyelitis vaccine may be refrozen if it thaws in storage or in transit, provided the temperature did not exceed 46°F (8°C). As many as ten freeze/thaw cycles are permissible for unopened vaccine, provided the entire duration of thaw does not exceed 4 hours and the temperature never exceeds 46°F (8°C). Once opened, vials of poliomyelitis vaccine must be kept refrigerated between doses and must be used within seven days.

If, for any reason, live virus vaccine is not returned to the refrigerator after thawing, discard it. Do not refreeze poliomyelitis vaccine after opening the vial. Use reconstituted vaccines for measles, rubella, and mumps as soon as possible after reconstitution. If the vaccine is not used within 8 hours, discard it. All reconstituted vaccine must be stored in a dark place at temperatures between 35.6°F and 46.4°F (2° to 8°C).

Specific vaccines have specific storage requirements and the product brochures should be consulted to ensure that these requirements are met. It would be impossible to detail all products here and even more difficult to anticipate the storage requirements of vaccines newly or soon to be released. It is imperative that the entire office staff be in-

---

* Adapted from guidelines compiled by the Monroe County Health Department, Rochester, New York, and the State Department of Health, Indiana, and many other sources, including product brochures. See *References.*

formed of the necessary storage procedures. A few that are currently recommended will be listed here.

Store influenza virus, typhoid, and cholera vaccines, and immune serum globulin (IG) at refrigerator temperatures between 35°F and 46°F. *Do not freeze these products* because biologic alteration can result in diminished potency. Smallpox vaccine, if used at all, should be stored below 0°C.

Once adequate storage has been ensured, the vaccine area or tray should contain appropriately sized syringes and needles and materials for sterilizing the skin prior to administration. Most physicians prefer to use individually packaged sterile units which, despite slightly increased costs, are extremely practical. Disposable plastic syringes are desirable and, in fact, are mandated for some biologics as indicated in the individual sections.

In addition to immunization paraphernalia, the area or tray should contain potent 1 : 1000 aqueous solution of epinephrine and an injectable and oral antihistamine. Adequately sized syringes should be available for administering these products in the event of an untoward anaphylactic or other allergic reaction. Since serum samples are sometimes needed, provision should be made in convenient fashion to have available the appropriate receptacles and labels as well as blood drawing equipment.

The area should have a comfortable table and chairs with adequate restraint apparatuses if such are needed. The physician should anticipate the specific needs for all ages of patients and should provide methods for rapid and convenient immunization application.

There should be some area for those patients who will need a waiting period after administration of a biologic. The area should be within sight lines of the physician and his assistants so that untoward reactions can be detected immediately and appropriate therapy carried out.

INSTRUCTION OF PERSONNEL

It is vital that all personnel involved in immunizations be acquainted with all of the above features of the immunization area and be adequately instructed in the administration, precautions, limitations, and side-effects of vaccine administration. Any person assigned to perform a portion of the immunization procedure should be told what to report back to the physician in the way of observed reactions or perceived contraindications to the vaccine that has been prescribed. Personnel should also be instructed in sterile technique and, if responsible for recording immunizations, should be told of the necessity for including the manufacturer, the lot number, and the expiration date for each dose administered. Such personnel should also be instructed in the method of informed consent being used and the reasons for it. If any part of this particular task is assigned to someone other than the physician, all of the principles discussed in Chapter 3 should be heeded.

PRACTICAL TECHNIQUES IN THE ADMINISTRATION OF VACCINES

Anyone administering any biologic product should be familiar with the recommended route of administration. In order to avoid untoward local or systemic effects and to ensure optimal effectiveness of the immunizing procedure, only the recommended route of administration should be used. Injectable vaccines are administered in an area as free as possible of opportunity for a local neural, vascular, or tissue injury. Although used frequently in the past, the upper outer quadrant of the buttocks should only rarely be used. *Preferred sites* for vaccination include the anterolateral aspect of the upper thigh and the deltoid muscle of the upper arm. These areas should be used whether the vaccine is to be administered subcutaneously or intramuscularly. The anterolateral aspect of the thigh will provide the largest muscle mass in most infants and is the preferred site for patients in that age group. As the child grows, the deltoid mass achieves sufficient size to offer a convenient site for intramuscular injection. An individual decision should be made in any case based on the volume of the injected material and the size of the muscle mass into which it is to be injected.

Subcutaneous injections may be administered at either site at any age, although most clinicians prefer to use the anterolateral thigh throughout infancy. Some rabies vaccines must be given in multiple doses; extension of the subcutaneous sites onto the abdominal surface may be desirable.

Intradermal injections are generally given on the volar surface of the forearm, using a small-gauge needle.

Intramuscular injections should be administered deep into the muscle mass. Most clinicians prefer to use the so-called "Z" method of injection. With this method, the skin and subcutaneous tissue are retracted laterally over injection site. Once the injection into the muscle mass is completed (some clinicians prefer to inject a small amount of air to clear the needle), the needle is withdrawn and the skin is allowed to retract back to its original position. This results in a discontinuous injection tract which helps to seal the intramuscular tract at the muscle-subcutaneous junction. This method is used to prevent the vaccine from seeping back into the subcutaneous tissue and thus prevents irritation and localized abscess formation.

Children should be well restrained before injection of a vaccine or other biologic. If more than one injection is given, different sites should be used. Prior to vaccination, the skin should be prepared with either isopropyl alcohol or an iodine-containing cleanser followed by isopropyl alcohol. It is important to remove the iodine-containing cleanser in order to avoid irritating the skin. I've seen several instances of severe iodine burns caused by pooling of the antiseptic against the skin secondary to failure to completely cleanse the area with isopropyl alcohol. Prior to administration, the plunger of the syringe should be pulled back slowly to ensure that a vessel has not been entered. If no blood appears in the syringe, the injection can proceed. If blood does appear, the entire needle and syringe should be withdrawn, discarded, and a new setup employed for administration.

Syringes and needles should preferably be disposable in order to minimize opportunity for bacterial contamination. A separate needle and syringe should be used for each immunization. Needles and syringes should be disposed of in specially labelled containers in order to prevent accidental inoculation or theft. There are devices for disconnecting the needle from the hub, thus destroying any opportunity for illicit use of the syringe afterwards.

If glass syringes are preferred, great care must be taken to ensure thorough cleansing and sterilization. The cleansing method should provide for removal of all possible antigen from the syringe, and the sterilizing equipment used should be at recommended temperatures for a sufficient period of time to ensure sterility prior to reuse.

For subcutaneous or intradermal injections, a 25-gauge needle, ⅝ inch long, is recommended. For intramuscular injections, a 20- or 22-gauge needle, 1 inch to 1¼ inches long, is recommended.

For administration of IG or other gamma globulins, a sufficiently large bore needle longer than 1 inch should be used. It is often necessary to use an 18-gauge needle for such administration. With gamma globulin, the injection must be placed deep in a muscle mass; the needle should be long enough to fully enter the muscle. The large bore may be necessary because of the viscous nature of the solution. It is especially important with gamma globulin preparations to employ the Z method in order to avoid subcutaneous leakage. Large volumes of gamma globulin should be injected into the buttocks. Great care must be exercised to place such injections in the upper outer quadrant well away from the sciatic nerve and blood vessels. All personnel should be thoroughly familiar with this technique and if inexperienced, should be instructed as to both the proper technique and the dangers of inserting the needle medially.

If it ever becomes necessary to inject both a vaccine and its corresponding gamma globulin, it is vital that a separate syringe and needle be used for each preparation and that they be injected at distant sites in order to avoid any opportunity for mixing and neutralization of the antigen by the antibody.

Again, all manufacturer's instructions should be followed precisely. In order to ensure both safety and effectiveness, no deviation from established procedures should be permitted.

RECORDING IMMUNIZATION DATA AND RECORDING AND REPORTING ADVERSE CONSEQUENCES

An immunization record should be prominently displayed in the chart of each pediatric patient. The record should include the date, type, manufacturer, lot number, and expiration date of each dose of vaccine. There should be space to indicate the site of vaccine administration, and to record any adverse reactions. This immunization record should be easily readable and all personnel should be able to immediately identify those patients lacking required immunizations.

If possible, some system should be developed by which the physician can survey his practice for individuals who lack specific immunizations. This is especially true as children grow older and such immunizations as rubella and measles become increasingly important. As of this writing, no universally acceptable system has been developed which can be recommended. Many physicians have adopted a tickler system in which patients are listed with the dates of their next anticipated recommended immunization. This list is kept separate from the patients' records and serves as a reminder to the entire office staff to notify the patients or parents when the vaccination is due. A few physicians have even developed a reminder system analogous to that widely employed by dentists to notify their patients by postcard of the need for specific immunizations.

Any adverse reaction should be adequately documented, and if significant, probably necessitates a visit to the physician. Care should be taken to record any abnormal physical finding as well as a careful history of the event. Following immediate therapy, the physician should notify the manufacturer and the local or state health department of any serious reaction. This is especially important for new vaccines for which the entire range of side-effects may not be known. Any significant reaction under these circumstances should be reported immediately.

In addition to recording the immunization date in a specific immunization record, the physician should record in his regular medical encounter note the immunizations prescribed and provide some indication of the informed consent procedure. If a written note is used, it should be entered into the record at an appropriate place (see Chapter 3).

INITIATING A NEW VACCINE INTO PRACTICE

Whenever a new product becomes available, the physician should become thoroughly familiar with the recommendations of the major advisory bodies as well as with the product brochure that accompanies the vaccine or biologic. Sources for such information are detailed in Chapter 3. Before the vaccine is given to any child in the practice, the physician should ensure that the entire office staff is familiar with the product and with any special considerations for its storage, reconstitution, or administration. Significant side-effects and contraindications and precautions should be reviewed with the staff in order that uniform devices and procedures are employed in patient contact. This will become increasingly important as products with different formulations and biologic characteristics and varying administration routes become available.

REFERENCES

American Academy of Pediatrics: *Report of the Committee on Infectious Disease* (Redbook), 19th ed., Evanston, 1981

Center for Disease Control. General recommendations on immunization, morbidity and mortality. Week Rep, 29: 76:81–83, 1980

Frankel HH: Potential effects of temperature on killed vaccines. New Engl J Med 301:159, 1979

Fulginiti VA: Immunization—theory and practices. Kelley V, Brennemann R (eds): Practice of Pediatrics, Baltimore, Harper & Row, 1981

How to give an intramuscular injection. Spectrum 0:50–54, 1964–65

Indiana State Board of Health: Communicable Disease Weekly Summary, September 27, 1977

Monroe County Health Department Bulletin, Rochester, New York, October 2, 1978

Roberts RB, Stark DCC: Sterile procedures in the doctor's office. Med Surg Rev 1:24–28, 1970

5

The Scheduling of Immunizations

Vincent A. Fulginiti

THE RATIONALE FOR "ROUTINE" SCHEDULES

The timing of most immunizations is based upon consideration of both the epidemiology of the disease and the immune responsiveness of the host. The final recommendation results from these considerations plus field trials that have demonstrated effectiveness.

For some diseases, certain periods of life are accompanied by increased risks. For example, pertussis is of particular danger to very young infants, whereas measles is less so. Rabies exposure is likely to occur among certain age groups based on occupation and recreational activities. Influenza may represent a severe risk to the elderly and less of a risk to the very young. In short, for each disease an epidemiologic pattern has been discerned that assists in defining an age-related risk. These epidemiologic patterns are often altered once a vaccine becomes available and is widely used. Thus, the physician should be aware of current epidemiologic patterns so that scheduling of immunizations can be adapted to the new circumstance.

Newborn and very young infants do not have the full immunologic capacity they will enjoy later in life. Certain diseases and treatments will result in altered immunologic capacity at any age, and finally, certain persons are immunodeficient, either totally or in part, altering their capacity to respond to vaccines as well as increasing their susceptibility to natural disease. As a result of these and similar factors, vaccine administration may be predicated upon the age and health of the patient. In each disease section, specific attention has been paid to most circumstances that influence immunization scheduling. We will confine ourselves to general considerations and integration of all immunizations into recommended schedules.

In general, very young infants do not respond maximally to many vaccines. In addition, if a transplacentally transmitted antibody is present, the agent or substance in the administered vaccine may be completely neutralized; this is especially true for live virus vaccines administered parenterally. However, when the epidemiology of disease is considered, it may be necessary to administer vaccine at an immunologically undesirable time in order to afford even partial protection if the patient is at risk. For example, in areas where pertussis is highly endemic, it may be necessary to initiate immunization in the newborn. This is done with the full knowledge that such patients don't react as well at that age as they will six months or so later. However, if the risk of pertussis is high for the very young infant, initiation of immunization may afford some protection and is therefore desirable. Such action, however, must be taken into account in the total immunization of that patient, in that extended doses or extra booster doses may be needed (see Chapter 7 on pertussis).

In some immunodeficient persons, susceptibility to natural disease may be heightened. Immunodeficiency may be congenital or may be secondary to disease or therapy. It is often impossible to predict the specific immune response to a given vaccine in such patients. Often, a vaccine is recommended for use despite this uncertainty. For example, pneumococcal polysaccharide vaccine is recommended for use in the antibody-deficient patient. This is predicated on the risk data which indicate that pneumococcal disease occurs at a higher frequency and at greater severity in such patients than in the general population. At the same time, the patient may not respond to pneumococcal polysaccharide vaccine with antibody synthesis. However, since it is uncertain whether a given patient will respond, use of the vaccine is recommended. Some patients will in fact be protected because the capacity to respond to this particular antigen is not lost. Physicians who give vaccines to such patients should recognize the inherent limitations and the limited potential benefits.

Thus, a given vaccine is intended to be administered to someone who is both capable of an appropriate immunologic response and who will probably benefit from the protection afforded by the vaccine. As we have seen, the appropriate balance often compromises optimal immunologic effect in order to achieve effective disease protection, even in part.

One additional factor in the selection of an immunization schedule is the demonstration of individual and group responses. If a single dose of a specific antigen evokes the desired response in an individual patient and if this individual response is reflected across the vast majority of the group to be immunized, then a single, nonrepeated dose is selected. Live measles, mumps, and rubella vaccines, for example, evoke regular, predictable responses at highly acceptable levels in both individual patients and groups.

On the other hand, a single dose of oral poliovirus (OPV) vaccine may produce an immune response to all three types of polioviruses in a given patient, but does not do so with sufficient regularity to rely upon a single feeding of the vaccine. If the entire group of 2-month-old infants is considered, the irregularity of response is magnified. Thus, for this vaccine, multiple administrations for the individual patient are intended to provide maximal coverage within the group, that is, the multiple administrations will eventually immunize more than 95% of the entire population. A single administration may achieve only 60+% for all three types of poliovirus contained in the vaccine.

For some antigens, a single dose results in a less-than-optimal total response. As a result, repetitive doses are used for primary immunization and periodic booster doses are given in order to maintain the desired level of immunologic response. Diphtheria, tetanus, and pertussis vaccines are examples. In general, most inactivated bacterial and viral vaccines and many vaccines containing products of infectious agents are included in this group.

"ROUTINE" OR RECOMMENDED INFANT SCHEDULES

The currently recommended schedule for immunization of a healthy child is shown in Table 5-1. As can be seen, diphtheria, tetanus, pertussis, polio, measles, mumps, and rubella vaccines are recommended for every infant. Diphtheria, tetanus, and pertussis are combined in a single injection (DTP) and poliovirus vaccine contains all three types of polioviruses. Measles, mumps, and rubella are now combined in a single vaccine (MMR) and are usually administered in this fashion.

There are several assumptions underlying the recommendations in Table 5-1. First, the recommended intervals are considered optimal given the dual considerations of the epidemiology of the disease and of the immunologic capacity of the recipient. One question that often arises is what procedure to follow if the child does not appear at the recommended times. For DTP and polio vaccines, one should continue the immunization as if the usual interval had occurred, that is, if the child received a DTP vaccination at 2 months of age and did not reappear until 6 months of age, the immunization schedule should be continued as if the interval were the same as indicated in the table. In fact,

TABLE 5-1.   Recommended Schedules for Infant Immunization and Routine Maintenance of Immunity*

Age	Vaccine(s)	Other
2 mo	DTP, OPV	
4 mo	DTP, OPV	
6 mo	DTP, (OPV)	
12 mo		Tuberculin test
15 mo	MMR	
18 mo	DTP, OPV	
Preschool (4– 6 yr)	DTP, OPV	
14– 16 yr	Td	

* As recommended by the American Academy of Pediatrics, Committee on Infectious Diseases.

DTP = diphtheria and tetanus toxoids, pertussis vaccine; OPV = trivalent, live, attenuated oral poliovirus vaccine (types 1– 3); MMR = live attenuated measles virus, mumps virus and rubella virus vaccines in combination; Tuberculin test = preferably Mantoux (0.1 ml PPD intermediate—5 TU); some prefer screening tests (see text and Chapter 17); Td = tetanus toxoid and diphtheria toxoid, adult type.

no interval is unacceptable today. One should not restart the immunization schedule, irrespective of the interval between doses.

Second, although rubella and mumps vaccines can be administered to a 12-month-old child and result in an antibody response, they are commonly administered to a 15-month-old child along with live measles virus (LMV) vaccine in a combined vaccine. Live measles virus vaccine should not be administered to a child under 15 months of age because of the possible presence of circulating maternally derived neutralizing antibody which will inhibit vaccine virus replication (see Chapter 10 on measles for details).

Third, two doses of OPV are recommended at 2 and 4 months of age for most areas of the United States. However, in areas where polio exposure is likely to occur, such as in the southwestern states bordering on Mexico, a third dose at 6 months is considered desirable by some, including myself. This dose is optional.

Fourth, a tuberculin test is indicated at 1 year of age. The principle here is to be sure that the patient is tuberculin negative prior to his receiving the live virus vaccines at 15 months of age. This is a controversial recommendation which the Academy of Pediatrics still adheres to, but which the Center for Disease Control (CDC) does not endorse. I believe that the tuberculin test should be performed prior to receipt of

TABLE 5-2. Recommended Schedules for Infants and Children Not Initially Immunized in Early Infancy

Time	Less than 7 Years Old	7 Years and Older
First visit	DTP, OPV, Tuberculin test	Td, OPV,* Tuberculin test
1 mo later	MMR	MMR
2 mo later	DTP, OPV	Td, OPV
4 mo later	DTP, (OPV)	—
8–14 mo later	—	Td, OPV
10–16 mo later (preschool)	DTP, OPV	—
Age 14–16 yr	Td	Td
Boosters	Td q 10 yr	Td q 10 yr

* No OPV for individuals 18 years or older; if exposure likely, use IPV.

DTP = Diphtheria and tetanus toxoids, pertussis vaccine; OPV = Trivalent, live, attenuated oral poliovirus vaccine (types 1, 2, 3); IPV = Inactivated poliovirus vaccine (types 1, 2, 3); MMR = Live attenuated measles virus, mumps virus and rubella virus vaccines in combination; Tuberculin test = Preferably Mantoux (0.1 ml PPD intermediate = 5 TU); some prefer screening tests (see text and Chapter 17); Td = Tetanus toxoid and diphtheria toxoid, adult type

measles, rubella, and mumps vaccines under usual circumstances (see Chapter 10).

Fifth, children more than 7 years old should not be given DTP. The pertussis component is dropped and the dose of diphtheria toxoid is reduced. The designation Td represents the adult type of tetanus-diphtheria toxoid and only this preparation should be employed in patients beyond 7 years of age. The dose of diphtheria toxoid is decreased to avoid undesirable local reactions.

Recommendations for children who fail to receive primary immunizations at the times recommended in Table 5-1 are listed in Table 5-2. As can be seen, significant changes in the order of vaccine administration are recommended principally to ensure that protection against measles, mumps, and rubella occurs as early as possible. An unimmunized child should not be given measles, mumps, and rubella virus vaccines until he is at least 15 months old.

Alterations in this schedule may become necessary depending upon local epidemiologic circumstances. For example, if there is a measles epidemic and an unimmunized child presents, it may be desirable to simply alter the order of immunizations and to give MMR or LMV alone before commencing the other immunizations.

It should also be noted that anyone 7 years of age or older should be given Td, not DTP or DT.

Finally, there is no upper age limit for administration of measles, mumps, and rubella vaccines. However, OPV should not be administered to anyone over age 18. As indicated earlier, pertussis vaccine is discontinued and diphtheria toxoid is reduced in quantity after age 7.

SCHEDULING IMMUNIZATIONS IN SPECIAL GROUPS

A variety of special circumstances may alter the usual recommendations for immunization. In the section that follows, individual circumstances are taken into account.

THE PATIENT WHO HAS LIMITED CONTACT WITH THE HEALTH CARE SYSTEM

In some circumstances, particularly when return of the patient is not assured, some physicians prefer to administer a large variety of antigens simultaneously; DTP, OPV, and MMR may be administered concomitantly in such cases. There should be a separate site of administration for each vaccine and separate syringes should be used for DTP and MMR. At present, relatively few patients have received this combination of nine antigens and therefore data are insufficient to make this a secure recommendation except in extenuating circumstances. What data are available suggest no immunologic interference and no cumulative adverse effects.

IMMUNIZATION OF PREMATURE INFANTS

The appropriate age for commencing immunizations in prematurely born infants is uncertain. Few data are available on which to base a firm recommendation. Commonly, gestational age is ignored and immunizations are begun at the usual chronologic age, such as at 2 months for DTP. The theoretic considerations behind this practice include: (1) the lack of significant amounts of potentially interfering, maternally derived, transplacental IgG; (2) the observation that newborn infants can produce IgM and IgG antibodies in response to a variety of antigens; and (3) the observation that full-term infants immunized shortly after birth have similar antibody levels to those immunized at a later time in infancy when both groups are given booster doses nine months to a year after the primary series.

Clearly premature infants have different qualitative and quantitative responses to many antigens than they will later in life. However, neonates can respond to or become sensitized to antigens such that subsequent booster doses produce anamnestic or secondary responses. This suggests adequate immunization following the primary series. However, the value of immunizing premature infants at the usual chronologic age is not established. Until data on the effectiveness of DTP, are developed its benefits are uncertain. It is incumbent upon the physician to ensure adequate follow up and the administration of a booster dose 9 to 12 months after completion of the primary series.

Oral poliovirus vaccine represents a special problem. Although preferably given to infants at 2 and 4 months of age in the usual schedule (Table 5-1), administration to an infant in a premature baby nursery or other hospital unit is undesirable. Contact infection of other infants is possible and could represent a hazard if the infants were susceptible to paralytic disease. Although this latter consideration is purely hypothetical, one can conceive that an extremely immature infant might be at increased risk of acquiring polioviruses that have passed through the intestine of the OPV-vaccinated infant.

Therefore, OPV immunization is not recommended for inpatients at the usual chronologic age; rather, the series can be begun with a first dose given on discharge from the hospital with arrangements made to complete the series.

Of course, if a prematurely born infant is at home, OPV can be administered at the usual chronologic age with the same rationale as discussed for DTP above.

IMMUNIZATION ON EXPOSURE TO DISEASE

In a few instances, exposed, susceptible persons may be actively immunized even during the incubation period of the disease. Postexposure immunization is the rule in rabies. Unimmunized persons bitten by or otherwise exposed to a rabid animal are given both human rabies immune globulin and rabies vaccine after the virus has been introduced into the host. With the currently available human diploid rabies vaccine, there is every expectation that the recipient will be protected from the disease.

Occasionally, a susceptible child is exposed to measles and the physician must choose between giving preventive doses of immune globulin (IG) or giving live virus vaccine. If the exposure occurred at an institution or group setting so that the exact date of the exposure is known, it is best to administer LMV vaccine to every susceptible person in that population. Live measles virus vaccine results in effective immunity within seven days, whereas the incubation period for natural measles averages 11 days. Experience has shown that this method is effective in preventing measles in the exposed susceptible child and in conferring long-term immunity against subsequent exposures.

In household exposures, the patient may have been exposed some days prior to notification, and administration of LMV vaccine in this situation is more problematic than in the institutional setting. Some experts nevertheless recommend administering LMV vaccine within 72 hours of exposure if this timing can be determined with reasonable accuracy. Many physicians prefer to administer a preventive dose of IG (0.25 ml/kg) and then to administer LMV vaccine three months later.

When the patient is an exposed susceptible infant less than a year old, either LMV or IG may be used. Most experts prefer to administer IG to prevent measles in such cases, with subsequent immunization once the child is 15 months old. However, if measles is endemic in the community and the child has not yet been exposed, LMV vaccine may be effective. Because one cannot distinguish between those with and those without transplacental antibodies, it is recommended that a second dose of LMV be given at 15 months of age to any infant who received a dose before then.

In both mumps and rubella exposures, susceptible patients cannot regularly be protected by live virus vaccine immunization. Giving live virus to a pregnant woman is contraindicated (see sections on rubella and mumps). In mumps exposures, it is common practice to administer live mumps virus (LMuV) vaccine to presumably susceptible patients in the hope that mumps will not result from the current exposure and that the immunization will ensure permanent immunity. The most common situation is that of a father whose child has mumps and it cannot be determined if the father is susceptible; under such circumstances, administration of LMuV vaccine is recommended, for the reasons already given.

CHILDREN IN INSTITUTIONS

Children living in custodial institutions sometimes have special disease risks and thus immunization practices must be altered. Among the diseases that may represent a risk to such groups of children are measles, mumps, hepatitis A and B, and varicella.

Mini-epidemics of measles may occur in institutions. Although the immune status of each resident should have been determined on admission by reference to physician documentation of illness or immunization, and LMV vaccine should have been administered to all susceptible children 15 months of age or older, this is often not done. Thus, the introduction of measles into such a setting necessitates the administration of LMV vaccine to all those who are susceptible (see above and Chapter 9 on measles).

Mini-epidemics of mumps may occur among institutionalized children. It is recommended that any child entering a residential facility be assayed for history of physician documented mumps infection or immunization. Any child with a negative or questionable history should be given LMuV vaccine soon after admission. If, on the other hand, this has not been done and mumps is introduced into the setting, no prophylactic method will effectively limit spread or inhibit disease. The best course of action would be to administer LMuV vaccine to exposed susceptible children in anticipation of their not being infected from the current contact and being protected in the future.

Influenza can be devastating in an institutional setting. This is particularly true if the reason for residential custodial care involves diseases of the respiratory or cardiovascular system or other conditions that expose the patients to increased risk. Rapid spread, high total exposure, and underlying disease may all result in severe illness affecting a large number of residents simultaneously or in close sequence. The best measure is programmed immunization with current strains of influenza vaccine timed to provide immunity well in advance of possible exposure (see Chapter 17 on influenza).

Varicella can involve a high percentage of susceptibles in a residential setting. This is among the most contagious of diseases and often affects in excess of 85% of exposed, susceptible contacts. Unless there is an underlying disease rendering the susceptibles prone to serious complication or death, no prophylactic measures are recommended. With high risk individuals, selective use of varicella-zoster immune globulin (VZIG) is warranted (see Chap. 24).

Both hepatitis A and hepatitis B may be transmitted in residential settings. Prophylaxis with either IG or hepatitis B immune globulin (HBIG) is recommended and is discussed fully in Chapters 23 and 24.

CHILDREN WITH NEUROLOGIC DISORDERS

Children with neurologic disorders pose a special problem in relation to immunization. In general, static neurologic disorders in which symptoms are unchanging do not contraindicate vaccine administration. For example, if the child has suffered an anoxic insult at birth and has residual cerebral palsy, there is no contraindication to any of the immunizations. However, if the neurologic disease is progressive, with changing symptomatology, then immunization is contraindicated. For example, a child who has progressive encephalitis should not receive routine immunizations, since the underlying process might be aggravated or the natural progression of the underlying disease might be blamed on the vaccine. Pertussis vaccine evokes special concerns and the reader is referred to the chapter on pertussis in which this is fully discussed.

Children who have had natural poliomyelitis might not be immune to the other types of poliovirus. Inactivated polio vaccine (IPV) is preferred in such individuals. One would wish to avoid OPV purely on theoretic grounds, since the patient has already demonstrated paralytic disease on exposure to one of the natural polio viruses.

CHILDREN WITH CHRONIC DISEASES

Recommended immunizations should be administered to children with specific chronic conditions that render them susceptible to the natural disease. Simultaneously, for some disease conditions, live virus vaccine may be contraindicated. Thus, the practice of immunization among children with chronic diseases is conditioned both on their susceptibility pattern and on the risk of the vaccine for that disease, and must be individualized.

Children with cardiorespiratory, allergic, metabolic, or neurologic disease of significant degree may be more susceptible to complications of influenza, and diligent use of influenza vaccine in such populations is recommended.

Asplenic children, secondary to removal or disease, might be more susceptible to serious pneumococcal infections. Also, children with nephrosis or B-cell deficiencies are similarly at risk. If these children are over 2 years of age, they should receive pneumococcal polysaccharide vaccine.

Occasionally a question arises concerning a specific child with a rare disorder as to the appropriateness of live virus vaccine administration. Unfortunately, there is usually little or no systematic experience in such disorders and the physician should seek guidance before administering the vaccine in question. In general, possible risks and benefits will be considered, taking into account known and theoretic immunologic components of the disease and known adverse reactions of the vaccine.

IMMUNODEFICIENT OR IMMUNOSUPPRESSED CHILDREN

Some generalizations are offered based on the actual experience of administering vaccines to immunodeficient or immunosuppressed children. However, for many patients and for most of the vaccines, theory is the only guide because adverse consequences have not been reported or experience with the vaccine in that disorder is not available. Furthermore, the specific immune deficiency may be unknown or undeterminable in a given child. One must then rely upon general and theoretic considerations.

Use of live virus vaccines of all types is contraindicated in congenital disorders of immune function. Fatal poliomyelitis, vaccinia infection, and measles have occurred in such children. If an inactivated vaccine is available for a given disease, such as IPV in poliomyelitis prophylaxis, then in general it is indicated and should be diligently administered to avoid the risk of natural disease. In other disorders, such as measles and varicella, only IGs are available for postexposure prophylaxis.

For the child who is receiving immunosuppressive therapy, several factors weigh in the final immunodeficiency that results. The underlying disease, the specific immunosuppressive modality and its dose, timing and repetitiveness, and the previous infectious disease and immunization history all contribute to the precise definition of immunocompetence, and therefore to the actual risk of an immunizing procedure. For most children, these factors may be imponderables and physicians are unable to define the precise defect in relation to the proposed vaccine. For this reason, blanket contraindication to the use of live virus vaccines is generally recommended. Again, inactivated vaccines and IG should be used as is appropriate.

Once immunosuppressive therapy is discontinued, particularly in children with leukemia in remission, it is common practice to administer the necessary live virus vaccines. The exact interval has not been determined with precision. Many physicians prefer to wait at least three months and some six months after cessation of chemotherapy before instituting live vaccine administration. This practice is based on the assumption that immunologic responsiveness has been restored and that the underlying disease for which the immunosuppressive therapy was prescribed is either in remission or control.

In both congenital and acquired immunodeficiencies, the use of any vaccine might not result in the desired response. Obviously, if the particular defect is specific to the expected response to vaccine, the patient will remain susceptible despite having received an appropriate vaccine in efficient fashion. To the extent feasible, assessment of specific antibody level and, if available, other acceptable specific immunologic tests such as cell-mediated immunity following immunization should be obtained to accurately access the state of immunity and to serve as a guide for future exposure or immunization.

ADOLESCENTS AND COLLEGE POPULATION

Among adolescents and the college population are those who: (1) were not immunized with some or all of the recommended vaccines; (2) received inadequate vaccines; (3) received appropriate vaccines at the wrong age; and (4) received incomplete immunization regimes. In addition, an unknown number may have been vaccinated with a technologically unsound method, but these patients are undetectable and therefore will not be further considered here. There is no simple solution to this complex group of problems.

Mass solutions have included school immunization plans with catchup programs, and college and military spot campaigns occasioned by specific disease outbreaks. Individual solutions are necessary and entail identification of the specific immune-disease status in a given person. As indicated earlier in this text, it is imperative that physicians adopt some method for identifying susceptible patients in their individual practices, and those physicians responsible for college aged, military, and other similar groups should also seek susceptible members of those populations.

Live measles, mumps, and rubella vaccines can be safely administered at any age. Live rubella vaccine poses a theoretic risk for the pregnant woman and its use in postpubertal female patients should follow the guidelines in the chapter on rubella. Pregnancy also contraindicates the use of any live virus vaccine on a routine basis; one exception is OPV, which may be administered if the risk of disease is greater than any theoretic risk from vaccine virus.

Those 18 years of age or older should receive IPV if protection is necessary. Live poliovirus vaccine should be avoided in all adults except under very special circumstances (see Chapter 12 on poliomyelitis).

PARENTS OF CHILDREN TO BE IMMUNIZED

With the single exception of OPV, immunization of an infant or child poses no substantial risk to susceptible parents, guardians, or other adults in the child's environment. Live oral polio vaccine poses a special problem. Susceptible adult contacts sustain a real but very remote risk of infection from poliovirus excreted in the infant's stool. In almost all instances, such infection is asymptomatic and immunizing. However, once for every 4 million doses of vaccine distributed, paralytic disease will result in an exposed susceptible contact, usually an adult. One does not wish any unnecessary delay or omission of infant polio immunization. At the same time, one wishes to minimize the risk to the adult contact which may include parents, older relatives, baby sitters, and others with prolonged exposure and opportunity for fecal oral transmission. Two acceptable courses of action are recommended: (1) administer OPV to the infant irrespective of the immune status of the adult contact; or (2) elicit a history of polio immunization status of parents and proceed accordingly. If a parent is a previous recipient of a partial course of OPV, simultaneously administer OPV to the susceptible adult; if he is a previous recipient of a partial course of IPV, give a booster dose of IPV to the susceptible adult and OPV no. 1 to the infant; if no previous immunizations have been received or if immunization status is unknown or uncertain, give two monthly doses of IPV to the susceptible adult and on the third monthly visit give IPV to the adult and OPV no. 1 to the infant. The remaining OPV dose or doses can then be administered at two-month intervals.

HEALTH PROFESSIONALS

Health-care workers may come into contact with children and adult patients with contagious diseases, and thus may be at increased risk of contracting such diseases when contrasted with the general population. In addition, they may transmit such diseases to the patients they care for. Among these infectious diseases are pertussis, measles, diphtheria, chicken pox, rubella, mumps, hepatitis, tuberculosis, and meningococcal infections. Susceptible persons in such categories should be appropriately immunized on a mandatory basis following the usual guidelines for each disease and vaccine.

Physicians, nurses, and other health-care workers in contact with children and young adult patients who may have preventable communicable diseases should not be an instrument for transmission of the disease to other patients in their environment. If they are not sufficiently motivated to protect themselves, then consideration for exposed patients should be paramount. Those for whom the risk is heightened include hospital workers in obstetrics and pediatrics, physicians and nurses working in pediatric and obstetrical offices and clinics, and all those working in health areas in which large numbers of pregnant women are encountered.

Separate discussion of immunization for these diseases is included in each disease section.

FOREIGN TRAVEL

We cannot anticipate all possible risks and governmental requirements for the international traveler. The best source for comprehensive information is the annually updated CDC booklet *Health Information for International Travel*. However, disease incidences change, as do regulations, and the traveler should check with local and state health departments for updated information prior to travel. Enough time should be allotted to allow immunization schedules to be completed in an efficient and safe fashion.

REFERENCES

American Academy of Pediatrics: Report of the Committee on Infectious Diseases (the Redbook), 19th ed. Evanston, 1981

Center for Disease Control: Pneumococcal polysaccharide vaccine. Morb Mort Week Rep 27:25–26, 31, 1978

Center for Disease Control: Measles and school immunization requirements—US 1978. Morb Mort Week Rep 27:303–304, 1978

Center for Disease Control: Rubella vaccine. Morb Mort Week Rep 27:451–454, 459, 1978

Center for Disease Control: Influenza vaccine. Morb Mort Week Rep 28:231–232, 237–239, 1979

Center for Disease Control: Poliomyelitis prevention. Morb Mort Week Rep 28:510–511, 517–520, 1979

Center for Disease Control: Varicella-Zoster immune globulin. Morb Mort Week Rep 28:589–590, 1979

Center for Disease Control: Immunization program for Indochinese refugees. Morb Mort Week Rep 29:38–39, 1980

Center for Disease Control: Mumps vaccine. Morb Mort Week Rep 29:87–88, 93–94, 1980

Center for Disease Control: Rabies prevention. Morb Mort Week Rep 29:265–272, 277–280, 1980

Harrison HR, Fulginiti VA: Bacterial immunizations. Am J Dis Child 134:184–193, 1980

Marcuse EK: Can we design a better immunization mousetrap? Pediatrics 63:501–502, 1979

Marks JS, Halpin TJ, Iriun JJ et al: Risk factors associated with failure to receive vaccinations. Pediatrics 64:304–309, 1979

McDaniel DB, Patton EW, Mather JA: Immunization activities of private-practice physicians. Pediatrics 56:504–507, 1975

Philips CF: Children out of step with immunization. Pediatrics 55:877, 1975

Stiehm ER: Standard and special human immune serum globulins as therapeutic agents. Pediatrics 63:301–320, 1979

6
Diphtheria

C. George Ray

DISEASE

Since the fourth century BC, disease caused by *Corynebacterium diphtheriae* has been recognized as one of the most frightening infections known to man. Even now it constitutes a serious threat and creates difficult problems in management and epidemiologic control. The problems of clinical diphtheria as related to invasive and toxigenic effects are outlined in the list below. Mechanical airway obstruction, toxemic shock syndromes, and toxigenic myocarditis are the major causes of death. The greatest risk factors include the toxigenic capabilities of the infecting strain of bacterium, the immune status of the host, and the site of primary involvement—patients with nasopharyngeal diphtheria, for example, have a greater chance of dying than do those with nasal or cutaneous infections. The potential seriousness of the problem is further underscored by the fact that the annual case-fatality rates for nasopharyngeal diphtheria in the United States have remained constant at approximately 10% over the period from 1920 to 1970, despite the advent of antibiotics and the increased sophistication of medical management (Fig. 6-1). Also, during the past decade there has been a resurgence in the incidence of reported infections, particularly in the Pacific Northwest and the southwestern United States. These observations suggest that reduction in cases as well as improved prognosis can be achieved only by adequate immunization and earlier clinical diagnosis.

Causes of Morbidity and Mortality in Diphtheria

Respiratory tract
  Pharyngotonsillitis with or without membranes
  *Laryngeal, tracheal membranes with respiratory obstruction

---
* Important potential causes of death

71

Cervical lymphadenitis and edema
Nasal diphtheria with serous or serosanguinous discharge
Otitis media, otitis externa
Conjunctivitis, other mucous membranes
Skin
    "Classic" tropical ulcer
    Nonspecific: impetigo, ecthyma or wound infection
Interstitial nephritis, with albuminuria
Endocarditis (rare)
Primary toxigenic manifestations
    *Systemic toxemia, thrombocytopenia, occasional disseminated
intravascular coagulation, shock
    *Myocarditis (may not be apparent until 7 to 30 days after onset
of infection)
    *Neurologic findings: Bulbar palsies (first and second week of
illness), polyneuritis (onset usually delayed by 3 to 6 wk)

Fig. 6-1. Diphtheria: reported case and death rates by year, United States, 1920– 1979. The incidence of diphtheria in the United States is low and continues to fall; case–fatality ratios of respiratory diphtheria have not changed significantly since 1920. (CDC, MMWR Annual Summary, 1979, 28:54, Sept 1980)

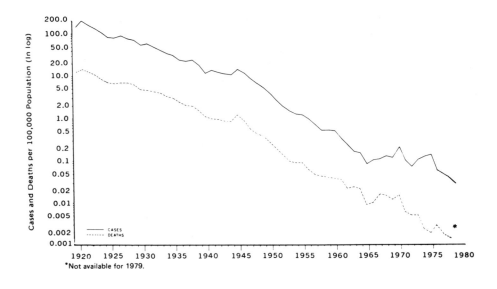

*Not available for 1979.

IMMUNIZING ANTIGEN

The antigen for immunization is formaldehyde-inactivated toxin (toxoid) produced by the PW-8 strain. The toxoid is available as either a fluid or in an aluminum-phosphate-adsorbed form. Because tests have shown that the adsorbed toxoids produce higher antitoxin titers for periods of longer time, the fluid vaccine is not recommended and will not be considered further.

Diphtheria toxoid is prepared singly or in combination with other antigens at two levels of potency. *D* is used to indicate the higher level of potency, and *d* the lower. A single dose of 0.5 ml of any of the *D* preparations is capable of stimulating an immune response; however, adequate immunity is achieved only with a complete primary series and appropriate booster doses. There is little evidence of the adequacy of primary immunization with *d* level vaccines; most experts believe that a full primary series with *d*-containing preparations will provide adequate initial protection and that a booster dose one year later will result in an appropriate secondary response. Circulating antitoxin levels of 0.02 units/ml or higher are considered protective.

The available preparations are as follows:

Diphtheria Toxoid, Adsorbed. This contains 7 IU to 25 IU of toxoid in 0.5 ml.

Diphtheria-Tetanus Toxoids, Adsorbed, Pediatric (DT). Each dose contains 7 IU to 25 IU of diphtheria toxoid plus tetanus toxoid. It is for use only in children under 7 years of age.

Tetanus-Diphtheria Toxoids, Adsorbed, Adult (Td). This preparation contains full amounts of tetanus toxoid but only 10% to 25% of the diphtheria toxoid (approximately 2 IU per dose) found in the DT or DTP preparations. It appears to be less reactogenic and of adequate immunogenicity for primary and booster immunization of those 7 years of age or older.

Diphtheria-Tetanus-Pertussis (DTP). This contains full doses of diphtheria and tetanus toxoids plus pertussis vaccine. It is intended only for immunization of infants and children less than 7 years of age.

RATIONALE FOR ACTIVE IMMUNIZATION

Corynebacterium diphtheriae causes disease in two ways. First, an invasive focus of infection is established in the respiratory tract, skin, ear, conjunctiva, or genital tract. In addition, lysogenic strains produce a potent protein exotoxin that facilitates cell destruction and local spread as well as systemic manifestations of disease. Strains that are nonlysogenic for the corynephages carrying the tox structural gene (nontoxogenic) are generally less virulent; however, they can sometimes cause local invasion with associated symptoms.

The exotoxin destroys many types of cells, but in humans the most significant effects are seen on the heart, the peripheral nervous system, and the kidney. Once the toxin has entered the cell, it can no longer be neutralized by antitoxin; such neutralization can only be certain when it is extracellular, and there is a question as to how effective the antitoxin is once the toxin is attached to cells.

The rationale for active immunization is to induce and maintain adequate levels of circulating antitoxin which will serve to neutralize exotoxin; this will in turn minimize the local spread of the organism in tissues and prevent the life-threatening systemic complications.

It must be emphasized that active immunization only confers *antitoxic* immunity which significantly reduces the risk of disease *per se*. Epidemiologic studies of diphtheria outbreaks have demonstrated that such immunity does not prevent acquisition of infection, usually as an asymptomatic carrier state or as occasional mild, localized disease. In order to effectively control spread of infection in outbreaks, asymptomatic as well as symptomatic carriers must be identified and treated with antimicrobial agents in order to eradicate the organism. It seems paradoxic that antimicrobial agents have a minor role in the prevention and treatment of active disease (they have no effect on the exotoxin) as compared with active or passive immunization, while the roles are somewhat reversed in the control of transmission of the organism.

Detecting nontoxigenic strains of *C diphtheriae* in a patient is somewhat reassuring, since these strains are usually associated with subclinical infection or mild, self-limited local disease. However, two observations may be cause for at least theoretic concern: (1) some patients harbor nontoxigenic and toxigenic organisms simultaneously and if the laboratory has not been careful to examine several different colonies, the latter group may be missed; (2) lysogenic conversion, whereby nontoxigenic organisms acquire the tox-positive corynephage, has been demonstrated *in vitro;* such conversion *in vivo* is possible but has not been demonstrated.

IMMUNITY

A full immunologic response necessitates a completed primary series and booster followed by periodic boosters throughout life in order to maintain adequate levels of circulating antitoxin. A crude method of assessing immunity is the Schick test, whereby 0.1 ml of purified diphtheria toxin (one fiftieth of the minimum lethal dose) dissolved in buffered human serum albumin (HSA) is injected intradermally on the volar surface of one forearm and a similar amount of purified diphtheria toxoid is injected into the other arm as a control. A positive reaction (erythema at the site of toxin injection beginning at 24 hours and progressing in intensity for about a week with no reaction at the control site) usually correlates with inadequate immunity, whereas a negative reaction at both sites is consistent with a protective level of circulating antitoxin of greater than 0.02 units/ml of serum. Transient reactions at both sites (pseudoreactions) or progressive reactions at both sites, more prolonged with the toxin injection (combined reaction), are much more difficult to interpret. The Schick test is considered a crude method of assessing immune status and is no longer routinely used in the U.S., nor is Schick test material available in many areas.

There are more precise *in vitro* methods of determining antitoxin levels and these have been applied to large-scale epidemiologic studies of immune status. Such tests are rarely used nor are they necessary for making decisions about the immunization needs of a particular patient, but the epidemiologic data derived from such testing have served to underscore the current deficiencies in our immunization programs. In one study, it was demonstrated that only 74% of healthy children who had received three immunizations in the past and 84% who had received four or more previous immunizations had what could be considered protective levels of circulating diphtheria antitoxin. A recent serosurvey of 183 urban adults was particularly disturbing—less than 25% of the entire group had adequate diphtheria antitoxic immunity!

Patients who have had clinical diphtheria rarely experience recurrence; nevertheless, recovery from infection does not necessarily confer immunity, and it is advisable to immunize such patients as appropriate for their age.

SCHEDULING OF DIPHTHERIA IMMUNIZATIONS

1. *Routine infant primary immunization.* The 0.5 ml DTP dose is given intramuscularly on four occasions, preferably beginning at 2 to 3 months of age. The first three doses are spaced at four- to eight-week intervals, the fourth dose approximately one year after the third. The usual schedule is 2, 4, 6, and 18 months of age. Another DTP booster is given at school entry, and then every ten years thereafter as Td (see Table 5-1, Chap. 5).
2. *Immunization of infants and children who fail to be immunized according to the routine schedule.* For children up to 7 years of age, DTP or DT may be used in the same schedule noted above.

If there is a lapse in the schedule, the immunizations are resumed without giving extra doses above the total of four in a
primary series (see Table 5-2, Chap. 5).

3. *Immunization of school children and adults.* For persons 7 years
of age or older, three 0.5 ml doses of Td should be given intramuscularly, the second dose four to eight weeks after the
first, and the third dose six months to one year after the second
(see Table 5-2, Chap. 5).

4. *Recall immunization.* Between 3 years and 7 years, either DT or
DTP may be used. After the seventh birthday, Td is given intramuscularly every ten years.

5. *Special circumstances.* When DTP has been used as the primary
immunizing preparation and severe systemic or neurologic
reactions have developed, this has usually been ascribed to the
pertussis antigen component of the vaccine (see Chap. 7 on pertussis). The usual action is to resume the series with DT instead.

Immunized close contacts of diphtheria should be given a booster
dose of diphtheria, DT, or Td toxoid, depending upon age, and unimmunized close contacts should begin a primary series immediately, as
was outlined. The specific management of cases and contacts will be
discussed in greater detail later in this chapter.

SIDE-EFFECTS AND ADVERSE REACTIONS

The general use of multiple antigen vaccines makes it difficult to
evaluate the side-effects of diphtheria toxoid. There are earlier data
derived from the use of this antigen alone, but the results are confused
by the fact that the older antigens were not prepared and purified in the
same way that they are now.

Acute reactions to DTP preparations in infants and children are usually blamed on the pertussis component. This is supported by the observations of Baraff and Cherry who compared the frequency of reactions to
DTP versus DT (Table 6-1). Serious side-effects with DT are uncommon
in infants, and more likely to occur in adult patients; this is why Td is
preferred for use in persons over 7 years of age. In persons with histories
suggesting severe local or systemic reactions to tetanus-toxoid-
containing preparations and who need diphtheria toxoid boosters because of close exposure, the diphtheria toxoid preparation alone may be
used.

The major side-effects of Td toxoids have been seen in adult patients;
in one recent study, as many as 57.8% reported at least one reaction,
including sore arm (42.7%), swelling at the site of injection (34.8%), and

TABLE 6-1. Vaccine Reactions: DTP vs DT

Type	Percent Reported	
	DTP	DT
Local reactions		
Redness	51.0	16.7
Swelling	56.3	16.7
Pain	49.7	18.9
More serious reactions		
Persistent screaming	5.9	2.2
Convulsions	0.2	0.0
Collapse	0.2	0.0

(Baraff LJ, Cherry JD: Nature and rates of adverse reactions associated with pertussis immunization. In Manclark CR, Hill JC (eds): International Symposium on Pertussis. DHEW Publication No. (NIH) 79-1830, 1979)

itching (24.2%). Serious side-effects, which were uncommon, include swelling of the arm below the elbow (1.1%), and abscess or cellulitis (0.7%).

An even more rare side-effect is the reported occurrence of acute hemolytic anemia in three infants following the second or third DTP injection. These patients had positive reactions to direct antiglobulin tests during the acute phase and the investigators suggested that a toxoid antigen-antibody reaction on the erythrocyte surfaces may have been involved in the pathogenesis. However, it was not clear which of the three vaccine components might have been involved in their illnesses. Urticarial reactions have also been noted.

SPECIFIC PRECAUTIONS

There are no specific precautions for use of the diphtheria toxoid component of the various vaccine combinations available. When DTP is used in a routine schedule, it is wise to postpone an injection if there is an intercurrent illness, particularly if the patient is febrile. The occasional local and rare systemic febrile reactions that occur with Td or DT immunization are generally considered to result from too-frequent use of tetanus toxoid with circulating antibody, which may contribute to an Arthus-type reaction. A major inconsistency between the use of combined preparations and immunologic fact is that immunity to tetanus can be readily maintained with boosters at ten-year intervals, whereas diphtheria immunity can be relied upon only if boosters have been given within four years of exposure.

The Moloney test has been used to determine whether a person is allergic to components of the toxoid. The rest involves the intradermal inoculation of 0.1 ml of a 1 : 100 dilution of fluid toxoid. A positive reaction is characterized by erythema and induration, reaching a maximum in 24 hours. This test is not recommended as a routine precaution—it is not considered reliable and the current highly purified toxoid makes such testing less essential.

PASSIVE IMMUNIZATION

Diphtheria antitoxin is only available in the form of equine hyperimmune serum (see Chap. 2 for details). It is primarily used for treating infections in patients who are unimmunized, who have questionable immunization histories, or who have known histories of inadequate immunization. The value of using antitoxin in partially immune or nonimmune asymptomatic carriers and close household contacts is debatable. Some authorities recommend the intramuscular administration of 3,000 units IM in nonimmune carriers, whereas others prefer only close observation with concurrent antimicrobial therapy to eradicate the carrier state.

Several facts must be considered when deciding whether to use antitoxin. First, the risk of fatal myocarditis or bulbar paralysis increases dramatically if there is a delay in treatment (fourfold or greater if the lapse is four days from the onset of illness). Therefore, a delay for the purpose of awaiting bacteriologic confirmation could prove lethal. Second, the toxigenic complications are most likely to occur with pharyngeal disease and are less likely with nasal or cutaneous lesions; however, there are risks associated with all of these. Furthermore, pharyngeal diphtheria may not always present with membranes or exudate; erythema, dysphagia, and a low-grade fever may be the only signs and symptoms. Third, the use of antitoxin also poses a considerable amount of difficulty and risk; approximately 10% of patients experience side-effects in the form of nonspecific febrile reactions or serum sickness syndromes. Anaphylaxis, although rare, is also a potential threat.

The quantity of antitoxin administered is determined quite arbitrarily, with a tendency to err toward using more than may actually be necessary. After appropriate skin testing, followed by conjunctival testing to detect hypersensitivity, follow these rough guidelines for antitoxin dosing: mild diphtheria (localized skin or nasal), 10,000 to 20,000 units; moderate disease (pharyngeal), 20,000 to 40,000 units; severe disease (systemic, multiple sites, delayed treatment), 50,000 to 100,000

TABLE 6-2. Desensitization With Dilute Diphtheria Horse-Serum Antitoxin*

Amount	Antitoxin dilution	Route
0.25 ml	1 : 100	SC
0.5 ml	1 : 100	SC
0.1 ml	Undiluted	SC
0.2 ml	Undiluted	SC
0.5 ml	Undiluted	IM

* The above amounts should be given at 20-minute intervals and if any reaction is observed, further attempts to administer antitoxin should be discontinued.
SC = subcutaneously; IM = intramuscularly

units. Give the total dose at one time, intravenously in 100 to 200 ml of normal saline over a period of 30 to 60 minutes. Some experts suggest giving half the dose intramuscularly and half intravenously; however, there is no evidence that this offers any advantages.

If skin or conjunctival testing indicates a risk of hypersensitivity, then carry out careful desensitization according to the protocol outlined in Table 6-2. Establish an intravenous drip first, and make sure a syringe containing 1 : 1000 aqueous epinephrine is available in the event of an anaphylactic reaction. Such a reaction may make it necessary to discontinue further attempts to administer antitoxin (see Chap. 2).

VACCINE, ANTITOXIN, AND ANTIBIOTICS IN CLINICAL DISEASE

Active Cases. The management of active cases includes antitoxin therapy as outlined above and antibiotics as follows:

Adult patients: Procaine penicillin, 600,000 units intramuscularly every 12 hours for ten days; or phenoxymethyl penicillin, 250 mg orally four times daily for seven to ten days; or erythromycin, 500 mg orally four times daily for seven days.

Children: Crystalline penicillin G, 300,000 units intravenously or intramuscularly every 6 hours for seven to ten days; or phenoxymethyl penicillin, 125 to 250 mg orally four times daily for seven to ten days; or erythromycin, 40 to 50 mg/kg/day orally in four divided doses for seven days.

Follow-up cultures are essential to assure eradication of the organisms.

Because active disease does not necessarily confer antitoxic immunity, active immunization should be planned to begin after the patient has recovered. The exact timing for this in the previously unimmunized patient treated with antitoxin is uncertain, but is probably appropriate three to four weeks after antitoxin has been given. The patient with an uncertain or known inadequate immunization series should be given a toxoid booster immediately, in the hope that a recall antibody response may develop early.

Asymptomatic Carriers and Close Household Contacts. After appropriate cultures have been obtained (including deep nasopharyngeal *and* pharyngeal swabs), antibiotics are used for at least seven days with follow-up cultures after treatment. The options for antibiotic prophylaxis include 600,000 units of benzathine penicillin G (particularly if poor compliance is expected) or oral penicillin or erythromycin as outlined for symptomatic cases. Diphtheria toxoid immunization series or boosters are commenced immediately with the patients being checked daily for at least seven days for the development of clinical signs and symptoms of diphtheria. The value of antitoxin therapy for nonimmune close contacts or carriers is debatable; however, when close surveillance is not possible, 3,000 units of antitoxin administered intramuscularly is suggested.

ISOLATION PRECAUTIONS

All active cases should be managed in the hospital with strict isolation precautions. It must be remembered that diphtheria can be spread through direct contact and through respiratory and fomite routes.

It is usually not feasible or necessary to isolate or otherwise strictly quarantine carriers; they can be treated at home but need careful clinical and bacteriologic follow up in cooperation with public health authorities.

REFERENCES

Crossley K, Irvine P, Warren JB et al: Tetanus and diphtheria immunity in urban Minnesota adults. JAMA 242:2298–2300, 1979

Dobie RA, Robey DN: Clinical features of diphtheria in the respiratory tract. JAMA 242:2197–2201, 1979

Haneberg B, Matre R, Winsnes R et al: Acute hemolytic anemia related to diphtheria-pertussis-tetanus vaccination. Acta Paediatr Scand 67:345–350, 1978

Koopman JS, Campbell J: The role of cutaneous diphtheria infections in a diphtheria epidemic. J Infect Dis 131:239–244, 1975

Marcuse EK, Grand MG: Diphtheria in San Antonio, Texas, 1970. JAMA 224:305–310, 1973

Middaugh JP: Side effects of diphtheria-tetanus toxoid in adults. Am J Pub Health 69:246–249, 1979

Miller LI, Older JJ, Drake J, Zimmerman S: Diphtheria immunization. Effect upon carriers and the control of outbreaks. Am J Dis Child 123:197–199, 1972

Munford RS, Ory HW, Brooks GF, Feldman RA: Diphtheria deaths in the United States, 1959–1970. JAMA 223:1890–1893, 1974

Nelson LA, Peri BA, Rieger CH et al: Immunity to diphtheria in an urban population. Pediatrics 61:703–710, 1978

Sheffield FW, Ironside AG, Abbott JD: Immunization of adults against diphtheria. Br Med J 2:249–250, 1978

Simmons LE, Abbott JD, Macaulay M et al: Diphtheria carriers in Manchester: Simultaneous infection with toxigenic and non–toxigenic mitis strains. Lancet 1:304–305, 1980

7
Pertussis

Vincent A. Fulginiti

DISEASE

Pertussis (whooping cough) is caused by infection with *Bordetella pertussis* (*Haemophilus pertussis*), a small, nonmotile, gram-negative bacillus. First described in 1906, pertussis is characterized by a biphasic clinical course followed by a convalescent period. Its primary manifestations are nonspecific respiratory symptoms (catarrhal period), building to a paroxysmal coughing period with a typical inspiratory whoop (paroxysmal stage), and followed by a gradual diminution of symptoms (convalescent phase) during which exacerbation can occur.

The disease affects all populations throughout the world; precise incidence, severity, and complications differ from place to place, within and across national and continental boundaries. Most serious disease occurs among infants, with 10% of all cases and 75% of all deaths occurring in the first year of life. In some places, pertussis occurs in very young infants lacking transplacental protection. Although older children can contract infection (a third of cases occur in children 7 years of age or older), the disease is milder with lessened morbidity and mortality. Even adults can be infected; a special problem exists for health-care personnel who may develop pertussis upon contact with clinical cases. (See Figure 7-1 for reported pertussis case rates in the United States from 1950 to 1979.)

Complications of pertussis include:

Superinfection. Pneumococci, staphylococci, and other bacteria can produce severe, even lethal pneumonia. *B. pertussis* itself can also produce a severe and progressive interstitial pneumonia. Pyogenic complications of pneumonia, from whatever cause, can ensue, with empyema and bronchiectasis prominent.

Hemorrhagic disease. Bleeding into the structures of the head, including the brain, can occur as a result of the pressures generated in the vascular system secondary to intense paroxysms of coughing. Further, coagulation may be interfered with, possibly resulting from the effects of endotoxin.

Central nervous system. Severe cerebral damage may result from hemorrhage, anoxia, alkalotic tetany (vomiting), and a toxic encephalopathy.

Miscellaneous. Atelectasis is common as is hyperaeration during the acute phase. Vomiting may be excessive and may lead to electrolyte and fluid imbalance. Nutrition may be suboptimal. Prolapse of the rectum, appearance of hernias, and ulceration of gingival structures may result from excessive paroxysms.

THE IMMUNIZING ANTIGEN

Pertussis vaccine is a chemically inactivated, whole bacterial suspension. Bacteria are grown as Phase I organisms killed with phenol or formalin. The final vaccine contains a preservative, usually an organic

Fig. 7-1. Pertussis (whooping cough): reported case rates by year, United States, 1950–1979. Although the annual incidence of reported pertussis cases declined markedly between 1950 and 1970, the reported case rate has remained fairly constant over the past 10 years. (CDC, MMWR Annual Summary, 1979, 28:54, Sept 1980)

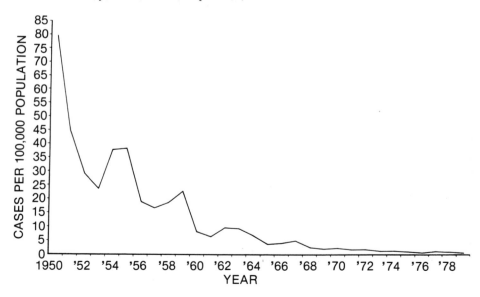

mercurial. Concentration is adjusted so that each 0.5 ml contains 4 protective units of pertussis antigen as judged by mouse-protection tests.

The specific antigen responsible for evoking the desirable immune response is not known. In general, the antibody tested is agglutinating but its protective effectiveness is uncertain.

An unlicensed product under study contains a chemically extracted pertussis antigen instead of whole bacilli. This preparation is designed to preserve antigenicity and protective effort and to reduce side-effects and adverse reactions. It is not commercially available.

RATIONALE FOR ACTIVE IMMUNIZATION AGAINST PERTUSSIS

Protection against pertussis is desirable because of the extensive morbidity and predictable mortality from the disease, particularly in young infants.

This disease is prevalent in the young, so immunization programs have been designed to provide protection as early as is immunologically feasible. The major reason for scheduling primary immunization with diphtheria-tetanus-pertussis vaccine (DTP) in the first months of life is to provide protection against pertussis.

Pertussis immunization has been curtailed in patients beyond 7 years of age. It is believed, although the data are few, that the risk of adverse reactions to pertussis vaccine increases in late childhood, thereby arguing against continued pertussis immunization. With today's knowledge, the early cessation of pertussis immunization must be viewed as arbitrary. A further reason for age-limited use of pertussis vaccine is the relative mildness of disease in older children and adult patients when contrasted with the morbidity and mortality in infants.

In recent years, localized epidemics of pertussis have been reported among adult contacts (family and health-care workers) of infants with pertussis. Some feel that physicians, nurses, and others likely to encounter pertussis should receive 0.25 ml booster doses of pertussis vaccine.

IMMUNITY AGAINST PERTUSSIS

Although several antigens have been characterized in *B. pertussis* and several antibodies identified in humans following exposure to these antigens, the precise mechanism of immunity is unknown. Almost total protection has been associated with high agglutinating antibody titers (more than 1 : 320) in humans and in monkeys. However, some protection (approximately 60%) occurs at serum antibody levels below this and has been recorded even in the absence of detectable antibodies. The role of other immune mechanisms such as cell-mediated immunity (CMI) has not been adequately explored.

Virtually complete immunity follows an attack of the natural disease, and recurrence of bacteriologically proven disease is rare. Protection following vaccine is relatively short-lived; booster doses are needed in order to maintain immunity. Complicating assessment of immunity is the pertussis syndrome caused by agents other than *B. pertussis.* Parapertussis has been estimated to account for as many as 2% of clinical cases attributed to pertussis. There is no cross-immunity between these organisms. Adenoviruses and other viral agents have been identified in pertussislike syndromes. Such infections confuse evaluation of the effectiveness of pertussis vaccine unless precise and definitive laboratory diagnosis is undertaken.

SCHEDULING OF PERTUSSIS IMMUNIZATION

ROUTINE INFANT PRIMARY IMMUNIZATION

Since pertussis morbidity and mortality are greatest in early infancy, routine immunization is usually begun at 2 months of age. The usual schedule comprises DTP at 2, 4, and 6 months of age at 0.5 ml per visit (4 protective units each; a total of 12 protective units). The primary series is completed with an additional 0.5 ml dose given 1 year after the last dose in the primary series of three.

IMMUNIZATION OF INFANTS AND CHILDREN NOT IMMUNIZED ACCORDING TO THE ROUTINE SCHEDULE

Protection against pertussis is ordinarily desirable through 7 years of age. Thus, two or three 0.5-ml doses spaced one to two months apart followed by a third dose a year later constitute adequate primary immunization (see Tables 5-1 and 5-2). As the child approaches 7 years of age, receipt of vaccine is predicated upon potential contact with infants rather than for primary protection of the patient. Thus, individual decisions must be made for the susceptible 6- or 7-year-old child who has never received vaccine, and must be based on family structure, babysitting arrangements, nursery school, and the like which may expose infants to the patient and vice versa. If such exposure is likely, pertussis protection is warranted.

IMMUNIZATION FOR ADOLESCENTS AND ADULTS

Ordinarily, pertussis vaccine is *not* administered to children beyond the 7th birthday. If pertussis is endemic in teenagers, then one may wish to continue booster doses beyond this age limit.

Health-care workers may be exposed to infants with pertussis and thus may experience the disease, often to a severe degree. Some experts advise *routine* administration of 0.25-ml booster doses to previously immunized adults likely to be exposed (*e.g.*, nurses and pediatric residents).

RECALL IMMUNIZATIONS

After completion of the routine primary series (at 2, 4, 6, and 18 months of age), a 0.5-ml booster dose is administered prior to school entry (at 4 to 7 years of age). Except as noted above, no further recall doses are recommended.

SPECIAL CIRCUMSTANCES

Two categories warrant comment. The first involves those who have had previous severe reactions. In such cases, no further pertussis vaccine should be administered. With less severe reactions (no central nervous system [CNS] symptoms), some clinicians prefer to give reduced doses (0.25 ml or 0.1 ml); if this route is selected, the *total* dose should equal 12 protective units (0.5 ml = 4 protective units).

The second category involves the neurologically handicapped child. If a child has a stable CNS disease (*e.g.*, stable hydrocephalus with unchanging manifestations), pertussis immunization should proceed as usual. If the CNS lesion is dynamic and evolving (*e.g.*, degenerative encephalopathy), *no* pertussis vaccine should be administered. The immunization reaction may exacerbate the disease or progression of the disease may be falsely attributed to the vaccine. Seizure disorders are a dilemma; on the one hand, one wishes to avoid adding a potential convulsion-evoking stimulus (vaccine), but on the other hand, pertussis itself may aggravate pre-existing convulsive disorders. In general, if the disorder is well controlled, one may proceed with pertussis immunization. If the disorder is severe or uncontrolled by medication, administration of pertussis vaccine is contraindicated. Some experts, some countries, and some organizations recommend that *no* pertussis vaccine be given to anyone with a personal or family history of convulsions. All advisory bodies in the United States do *not* advocate elimination of pertussis vaccine because of a family or personal history of seizures.

Obviously, these considerations ordinarily preclude early infant immunization until one has had an opportunity to evaluate the status of the convulsive disorder and the response to therapy.

SIDE-EFFECTS

The majority of observations indicate a high frequency of local induration and inflammation at the site of pertussis vaccination; as many as 70% of recipients may experience some degree of local irritation plus fever. In rare cases, local necrosis may occur, resulting in the so-called sterile abscess or cyst which may necessitate surgical drainage. Even more rarely, such areas can become bacterially infected.

Uncomplicated fever is considered a side-effect and occurs frequently. The usual complex of side-effects comprises a sore nodule plus slight or modest elevation in temperature associated with mild irritability and anorexia; these side-effects generally develop 2 to 6 hours after receipt of the vaccine and last less than 24 hours. There is no evidence that prophylactic use of antipyretics or sedatives has any beneficial effect.

ADVERSE REACTIONS

A variety of serious reactions to pertussis vaccine have been reported. There is disagreement as to their frequency, their etiologic connection with pertussis vaccine, and their significance *vis-à-vis* routine use of pertussis vaccine.

ANAPHYLAXIS

A type-I (IgE-mediated) response to an offending allergen, anaphylaxis has been associated temporally with vaccines containing pertussis as a component. Local anaphylaxis (urticaria) has rarely been reported following DTP or pertussis vaccine. It is usually benign and self-limited, necessitating only symptomatic measures.

Systemic anaphylaxis has been attributed to pertussis vaccination. The precise link and the incidence are controversial. Usually, a temporal association is noted (minutes to 12 hours) after receipt of the vaccine, but definitive studies are rarely performed or reported. Shock, sudden collapse, cardiorespiratory arrest, and sudden infant death all have been associated with pertussis vaccine. It has been estimated that the incidence is one per one million doses with a mortality of less than one per one million doses. Some have compared these human situations to the adrenergic blockade observed in the mouse following pertussis vaccine.

INADVERTENT ADMINISTRATION BY INCORRECT ROUTE

There may be a severe local reaction if the vaccine is administered subcutaneously or intradermally. Such a rare event is preventable by paying meticulous attention to the details of intramuscular administration (see Chap. 4).

Systemic collapse may follow intravenous injection, mimicking anaphylaxis (see Chap. 4).

THROMBOCYTOPENIA

Rarely noted and possibly unrelated to pertussis vaccine, thrombocytopenia may occur one to two weeks following vaccination. Since there are many other possible causes, it is often difficult to link this condition directly to pertussis vaccination.

CENTRAL NERVOUS SYSTEM REACTIONS

This section will deal with an assortment of conditions occurring in temporal association with pertussis vaccine, not all of which are clearly defined or necessarily proven to be causally related.

Grand Mal Seizures. Grand mal seizures, either single or multiple, may follow pertussis vaccine administration; most (50% to 75%) occur within 24 hours but some investigators have described seizures occurring up to two weeks later that were believed to be related to the vaccine. Most occur during the primary series and are uncommon after booster doses. Most convulsions (up to 80%) are accompanied by fever, suggesting a causative relationship in at least some of them, especially in the single episodes.

Seizures in themselves do not imply prolonged disability. If unassociated with encephalopathy, the prognosis is excellent; prolonged seizures, status epilepticus, or continued seizure disorders are rare. Generally, symptomatic therapy and anticonvulsant medication used acutely suffice.

There is some evidence that certain children might be predisposed to convulsions after pertussis vaccination; some investigators believe that a personal or family history of febrile or other convulsions, or a history of convulsions following previous doses of pertussis vaccine, make subsequent susceptibility more likely.

Screaming Episodes. Many infants cry and fret after pertussis vaccination; a few adopt a pattern of consistent crying for periods of an hour or longer; the crying is often of unusual pitch and intensity and the baby is inconsolable. This syndrome of screaming is believed to be encephalopathic in origin but there is no direct evidence such as cells in spinal fluid or electroencephalographic changes to support this clinical contention.

Children who experience such episodes are to be considered as having CNS complications and further pertussis vaccine should not be administered.

Encephalitic and Encephalopathy Syndromes. Alteration in level of consciousness, convulsions, excessive irritability, focal neuromuscular signs, and meningeal irritation constitute a group of clinical manifestations that may be considered the result of cerebral irritation and inflammation. Pertussis vaccine has been linked with such manifestations and terms such as "pertussis vaccine encephalopathy" are used to describe the association.

In 1948, Byers and Mall described encephalitis after pertussis vaccine. Only one case with autopsy examination was presented and complexities in interpretation of preexistent disease and inexplicable diagnostic findings resulted in uncertainty as to the precise nature of the linkage with pertussis vaccine. Since that time, many investigators have attempted to assess the linkage and the risk, with widely divergent results. These efforts may be summarized as follows. First, most observers accept onset of symptoms between 24 and 48 hours after pertussis vaccination as putative evidence of an etiologic link. Second, the age groups in which these CNS syndromes occur are also associated with causes of encephalitis, encephalopathy, and aseptic meningitis caused by a variety of conditions *other than* pertussis vaccine. Few observers have attempted to measure the background and contrast it with frequency following pertussis vaccination. Even fewer have exhaustively investigated individual cases for other causes.

Third, the rates of these syndromes vary so greatly as to be meaningless. Strom reported an incidence in Sweden in the 1960s of approximately 1 per 6000, a rate with which most disagree. Edsall has concluded that a range of 1 per 100,000 to 1 per 1 million is closer to the truth. Pollack found no cases among 80,000 vaccinees studied prospectively. British studies have shown no cases following 157,000 doses of vaccine. A 1977 British commission estimated risk of brain damage at 1 per 300,000 immunizations.

Critical to our discussion of side-effects and adverse reactions are the precise risks of any of these occurring among children receiving DTP, the most widely used preparation. Baraff and Cherry are currently investigating, in prospective fashion, the incidence of each of the above reactions in a group of infants receiving DTP in contrast to a smaller group receiving just diphtheria-tetanus toxoid (DT). Preliminary results of their study include the finding that minor local reactions consisting of redness, swelling, and pain occurred in about 50% of DTP recipients, compared with only about 18% of the DT recipients; fever was seen in 48% of patients given DTP, but in only 10% of those receiving DT. Drowsiness and fretfulness were experienced by 31% and 56%, respectively, of DTP recipients, compared with 18% and 20% of the DT recipients. Persistent crying for an hour or longer was reported in 5.9% of DTP recipients, as opposed to 2.2% of DT recipients. Convulsions and collapse each occurred in 0.2% of the DTP group, but in none of the DT group. Of four patients with convulsions, two were febrile at the time of their seizures, but all four were normal within 48 hours after being immunized. All four patients experiencing collapse were subsequently found to be normal.

SPECIFIC PRECAUTIONS AND CONTRAINDICATIONS

Pertussis vaccine should not be given to anyone who has had a severe reaction following a previous dose. The definition of severe reactions differs from expert to expert. What is meant here includes:

Previous convulsion

Previous persistent screaming episode

Any reaction with a "hard" CNS component (*i.e.,* any physical sign or well-described historic event suggesting CNS manifestation

Previous collapse or anaphylaxis

Occurrence of thrombocytopenia

Excessive fever (greater than 105°F or sustained fever at lower level)

A considered judgment should be made about children who have had seizures of a CNS disorder (as discussed previously). These conditions should not be considered contraindications *per se;* instead, they should emphasize the need for caution and a risk-benefit decision should be made for each child and each dose.

Precaution is urged when contemplating immunization of healthy persons older than 7 years of age. With clear-cut indications, as discussed earlier, 0.25 ml should be administered as a booster, or as a new dose if the patient has been immunized but is less than 7 years old.

PASSIVE IMMUNIZATION

The only product previously available for use in preventing or treating pertussis by passive means was pertussis immune globulin (human). It was prepared by hyperimmunization of adults with Phase I pertussis vaccine and was a characteristic human gamma globulin (see Chap. 24). There were no conclusive studies of its effectiveness; in fact, several controlled studies showed no benefit, either prophylactically or therapeutically. Therefore, in 1980, it was removed from commercial distribution and is no longer available.

The use of immune globulin is not indicated in pertussis prophylaxis or therapy.

Although unproven at present, some recommend that erythromycin therapy be used to prevent pertussis in exposed, susceptible infants, and that either ampicillin or erythromycin be used to decrease the period and intensity of bacterial shedding in infants with the disease and thus help to reduce spread of the organism. Antimicrobial therapy does not shorten the course of the disease or other symptoms.

REFERENCES

Altemeier VA, Ayoub EM: Erythromycin prophylaxis for pertussis. Pediatrics 59:623–625, 1977

Balagtas RC, Nelson KE, Levin S et al: Treatment of pertussis with pertussis immune globulin. J Pediatr 79:203–208, 1971

Baraff LJ, Cherry JD: Nature and rates of adverse reactions associated with pertussis immunization. J Pediatr 79:291–296, 1971

Center for Disease Control: Pertussis—Georgia. Morb Mort Week Rep 26:307–308, 1977

Editorial: Whooping cough vacillation. Lancet 2:71–72, 1977

Joint Committee of Vaccination and Immunization: Whooping Cough Vaccination. London Department of Health and Social Security, 1977

Kendrick P: Can whooping cough be eradicated? J Infect Dis 132:707–712, 1975

Kurt TL, Yeager AS, Guinette S et al: Spread of pertussis by hospital staff. JAMA 221:264–267, 1972

Linnemann EC, Partin JC, Perlstein PH et al: Pertussis: Persistent problems. J Pediatr 85:589–591, 1974

Malleson PN, Bennett JC: Whooping cough admissions to a paediatric hospital over ten years. Lancet 1:237–239, 1977

Mortimer EA Jr: Pertussis immunization: Problems, perspectives, prospects. Hosp Pract 15(10):103–118, 1980

Mortimer EA Jr, Jones PR: Pertussis vaccine in the United States: The benefit-risk ratio. In Manclark CR, Hill JC (eds) International Symposium on Pertussis, pp 250–255. Washington, D.C., U.S. Government Printing Office, 1979

Nelson JD: The changing epidemiology of pertussis in young infants. Am J Dis Child 132:371–373, 1978

Preston NW: Type-specific immunity against whooping cough. Br Med J 2:724–727, 1963

Provenzano RW, Wetterlow LH, Ipsen J: Pertussis immunization in pediatric practice and in public health. New Engl J Med 261:473–478, 1959

Provenzano RW, Wettelow LH, Sullivan CL: Immunization and antibody response in the newborn infant 1: Pertussis immunization within twenty-four hours of birth. New Engl J Med 273:959–963, 1965

Rulenkampff M, Schwartzman JS, Wilson J: Neurological complications of pertussis inoculation. Arch Dis Child 49:46–49, 1974

Sako W: Early immunization against pertussis with alum precipitated antigen. JAMA 127:379–381, 1945

Stuart-Harris CH: Experiences of pertussis in the United Kingdom. In Manclark CR, Hill JC (eds) International Symposium on Pertussis, pp 256–261. Washington, D.C., U.S. Government Printing Office, 1979

Weil C, Riley HD, Lapin JH: Extracted pertussis antigen. Am J Dis Child 106:210–215, 1963

Wilkins J, Williams FF, Wehrle PF et al: Agglutination response to pertussis vaccine. J Pediatr 79:197–201, 1971

8
Tetanus

H. Robert Harrison

DISEASE

Tetanus is caused by *Clostridium tetani,* an anaerobic, spore-forming, gram-positive rod. The bacterium is ubiquitous in nature and in the feces of animals and humans. It exists as an extremely resistant spore. Customary methods of inactivation have varying effects on spore-containing material. Autoclaving at 115°C for 15 minutes is reliable whereas boiling is not. The most reliable antiseptics are oxidants such as hydrogen peroxide. In nature, the concentration of spores in soil depends upon the amount of fecal contamination from artificial manure, humans, or animals. Approximately 25% of healthy people carry *Cl. tetani* in their intestinal tracts.

In tetanus, spores are introduced into an area of injury and can convert to the toxin-producing vegetative organism. This conversion is dependent on numerous factors including the establishment of an anaerobic environment and the presence of tissue damage. All the clinical features of tetanus are caused by the soluble exotoxin, tetanospasmin, which is produced by the vegetative organism within the wound. The organism itself causes no disease. Tetanospasmin is a protein with a molecular weight of 150,000, probably composed of two nonidentical polypeptide chains with molecular weights of 100,000 and 50,000, respectively. The heavy chain is thought to contain the specific binding site for a cell surface ganglioside on cells of the central nervous system (CNS). The cell receptor for toxin may be structurally similar to the receptor for thyroid-stimulating hormone (TSH) on thyroid cells. The exact mechanism of toxic action is unknown, although it appears to

induce hyperexcitability of motor neurons by interfering presynapti-
cally with release of an inhibitory transmittor.

Clinical tetanus has been reported to occur after exposure to organisms under the following major circumstances, although ultimately
any break in the skin is a potential portal for infection:

Wounds, either trivial or obvious. Half the cases of tetanus in the
U.S. in recent years have occurred after minor wounds for which no
medical attention was sought. Often, no wound is found at presentation with disease. Among these, tetanus-prone wounds may be defined
as severe trauma, burns, penetrating wounds, or any other trauma
associated with potential *Cl. tetani* contamination, such as animal
injuries, bites, multiple scratches, and kicks from horses. In addition,
wounds left untreated for more than 24 hours are considered
tetanus-prone. All such wounds, if sustained in an environment rich in
spores, such as barnyards, stables, or similar feces-contaminated
areas, are at particular risk. Furthermore, wounds that predispose to
anaerobic conditions, such as crush injuries, frostbite, or other
devascularization-type injuries, are also at high risk.

Following insect bites or stings.

In contaminated operative sites, particularly in relation to the
gastrointestinal (GI) tract. Devitalized, crushed, or injured bowel and
peritoneum are ideal anaerobic environments in which the patient's
normal fecal burden of *Cl. tetani* may flourish and produce toxin.
Furthermore, postoperative extraintestinal or extraabdominal devas-
cularizing injuries may become infected with the host's flora.

In improperly performed abortions or in puerperal infection in
normal childbirth. The uterine cavity is also an ideal anaerobic environment for *Cl. tetani*.

As neonatal tetanus, usually through contamination of the umbilical stump. This disease has all but disappeared in the U.S. The
patients are primarily infants born at home to unimmunized mothers
and the infection occurs through the use of unsterile methods.
Neonatal tetanus is still a major problem in several developing countries where aseptic delivery is not possible. It is also customary to
"treat" the umbilical stump with a variety of unsterile materials such
as soil and dung which may contain *Cl. tetani* spores.

Contaminated injections, particularly in narcotics abusers; the
quinine with which heroin is often cut may predispose to anaerobic
conditions in abscesses caused by subcutaneous administration.

Approximately 60 to 300 cases of tetanus occur annually in the U.S.
(Fig. 8-1), with no particular geographic localization. This finding is
consistent with the widespread prevalence of spores. Interestingly, the
incidence of disease and the case-to-fatality ratio for Caucasians in the

U.S. are much lower than in other races. (See Figure 8-2 for reported cases by age group.)

The overall mortality rate for tetanus is 45% to 55%, with the majority of deaths occurring in neonates and in adult patients over 50 years of age. There are three clinical forms of tetanus: generalized, cephalic, and local. Generalized tetanus is the most common type; two subtypes, neonatal tetanus and tetanus in heroin addicts, have particularly poor prognoses. Localized tetanus, which is manifested by persistent unyielding rigidity in the muscle groups adjacent to the injury, is generally mild, with a fatality rate of about 1%. It may progress to generalized disease. Cephalic tetanus, an unusual form following head injuries or otitis media, is characterized by numerous cranial nerve palsies and has a very poor prognosis.

PRINCIPLES OF IMMUNITY

There is no natural immunity to tetanus. Clinical immunity depends upon the presence of circulating antibody to tetanospasmin prior to fixation of the toxin to its ganglioside binding site. The strategy of

Fig. 8-1. Tetanus: reported case rates by year, United States, 1950–1979. The incidence of tetanus has been relatively constant for the last 5 years, probably because immunization rates for high-risk groups (persons over the age of 50 years and neonates) have not increased significantly. (CDC, MMWR Annual Summary, 1979, 28:54, Sept 1980)

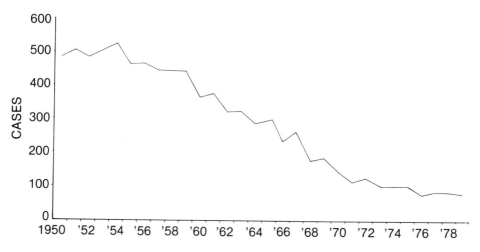

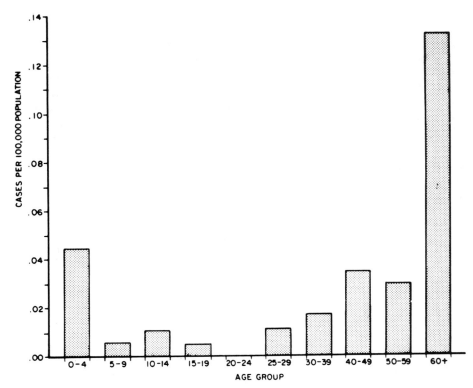

Fig. 8-2. Tetanus: reported case rates by age group, United States, 1979. (CDC, MMWR Annual Summary, 1979, 28:54, Sept 1980)

immunization is to provide prophylaxis through active stimulation of antibody well in advance, passive transfer of antibody at the time of exposure, or a combination of both.

Tetanus toxoid is formaldehyde-denatured tetanospasmin, a potent antigen with minimal toxicity. It is probably the most effective antigen used in immunization practice. Active immunization results in production of antitoxin antibodies rendering the patient immune to the binding and action of tetanospasmin. The rationale for infant immunization is to provide effective life-long protection with minimal risk against a ubiquitous and potentially lethal infection that may be encountered at any age.

Passive immunization is accomplished with human tetanus immune globulin (TIG), 250 units intramuscularly (IM). A dose of 4 to 5 units/kg provides a plasma level of 0.01 to 0.02 units/ml for four weeks or longer. There is no indication for use of horse serum in the U.S., but in some parts of the world TIG is not available and animal serum must be used. Passive immunization is employed only in special situations, to be discussed. The accepted protective level of antibody (actively or passively acquired) is 0.01 units/ml.

TETANUS VACCINES

Tetanus toxoid is available as an aluminum-phosphate-adsorbed vaccine or as a fluid vaccine. The fluid toxoid has been used only for booster doses when rapid protection is needed, but it induces antibody response of a much shorter duration. It is not recommended for use. Adsorbed vaccine (and not the fluid form) is antigenic in the presence of passively received antibody and is the only preparation recommended for primary immunization and for booster doses.

The adsorbed toxoid form is available as, a single antigen, as a triple antigen (diphtheria-tetanus-pertussis [DTP]), as the double antigens, diphtheria and tetanus toxoids adsorbed, pediatric (DT); and as tetanus and diphtheria toxoids, adsorbed, adult type (Td). The Td type contains a smaller dose of diphtheria toxoid than does DT and is used in those more than 7 years old for recall and in adult patients not previously immunized. The amount of tetanus toxoid is constant in all combined products.

SCHEDULING OF IMMUNIZATION

Three schedules for tetanus immunizations have been designed.

ROUTINE IMMUNIZATION

Children 2 months to 7 years of age should be given three DTP immunizations intramuscularly at six to eight week intervals, with a fourth injection one year after the third dose.

CHILDREN OVER 7 YEARS OF AGE AND ADULT PATIENTS NOT PREVIOUSLY IMMUNIZED

Two doses of Td vaccine should be given intramuscularly two months apart, with a third dose six to 12 months later. It should be noted that the first dose produces little or no rise in antibody titer; levels increase after the second and subsequent doses.

The decay rate of endogenous tetanus antitoxin is low in both children and adult patients. Furthermore, there is a strong correlation between reactions to booster doses and the patient's circulating antitoxin levels. A study performed by Peebles and colleagues in 143 pediatric patients demonstrated that none who had received four or more injections (a routine pediatric series) failed to maintain a protective antitoxin level for any measured interval. Furthermore, the interval of protection after four or more doses is longer than 12 years from the last dose with a confidence level of 99.9%. Consequently, special tetanus boosters on admission to camps, schools, and colleges, and emergency injections at times of injury have been abandoned when there is a valid history of routine immunization.

TETANUS-PRONE INJURIES

Tetanus-immune globulin (TIG) should be administered regardless of current booster status. When a previously immunized patient needs a booster, the immune globulin and a booster dose of toxoid are given at separate sites. In unimmunized individuals, primary immunization is begun in addition to TIG administration. Care should be taken to ensure completion of the series in order to avoid need for future TIG.

SIDE-EFFECTS AND ADVERSE REACTIONS

Reaction to tetanus toxoid administration may be categorized as generalized anaphylactoid (acute urticaria, angioneurotic edema, dyspnea, shock), local Arthus-type, and local delayed hypersensitivity-type. All reactions are uncommon in children.

Anaphylactic reactions to toxoid are very rare. The early cases were reported in large-scale armed services immunization programs conducted during World War II. Approximately one in 2000 U.S. Army recruits experienced flushing, itching, local and general urticaria, lip and eyelid edema, and occasionally dyspnea. Many of these reactions were associated with peptones used to prepare the vaccine. The reaction rate fell to one in 10,000 in adults when the use of these peptones was discontinued.

Arthus reactions are much more common; they are an exaggerated local response (swelling, erythema, occasionally necrosis) to the repeated injection of foreign protein. These reactions are allergic manifestations resulting from the union of toxoid and circulating antitoxin in the tissue at the injection site. The severity of this type of reaction is strongly correlated with the level of circulating antitoxin at the time of inoculation. Erythema and swelling have been observed in 29% and 74%, respectively, of 15- and 16-year-olds given routine booster toxoid doses.

REFERENCES

Brooks VB, Curtis DR, Freles JC: Mode of action of tetanus toxin. Nature 175:120–121, 1955

Edwall G: The current state of tetanus immunization. Hosp Pract 6: 57–66, 1971

Fultborpe AJ: The influence of mineral carriers on the simultaneous active and passive immunization of guinea-pigs against tetanus. J Hygiene 63:243–262, 1965

Rothstein RJ, Baker FJ: Tetanus: Prevention and treatment. JAMA 240:675–676, 1978

Scheibel I, Bentzon MW, Christensen PF et al: Duration of immunity to diphtheria and tetanus after active immunization. Acta Pathol Microbiol Scand 67:380–392, 1966

Steigman AJ: Abuse of tetanus toxoid. J Pediatr 72:753–754, 1968

Turner TB, Velasco-Joven EA, Prudovsky S: Studies of the prophylaxis and treatment of tetanus: I. Studies pertaining to treatment. Bull Johns Hopkins Hosp 102:71–84, 1958

Weinstein L: Tetanus. New Engl J Med 298:1293–1296, 1973

9
Rubella

E. Russell Alexander

DISEASE

Rubella is a mild disease of children and young adults caused by the rubella virus, first isolated in 1964. The usual clinical manifestations include a maculopapular rash that usually starts on the face and spreads to the trunk and extremities. The rash rarely lasts longer than three days. Generalized lymphoadenopathy precedes the rash, sometimes by as much as a week. Particularly characteristic are tender retroauricular, posterior cervical, and occipital adenopathy. At least half of all cases occur without rash and lymphoadenopathy may be the only recognizable manifestation. Constitutional symptoms are mild and fever is usually less than 101°F, rarely lasting longer than the rash. Arthritis and arthralgia, uncommon in children, are frequently noted in young adults, particularly in women. Encephalitis and neuritis are rare complications; the former occurs only once in 5000 cases. Thrombocytopenic purpura is also a rare complication of rubella. Before the use of vaccine, rubella occurred most frequently in the school age child (peak, 5 to 9 years). Figure 9-1 outlines the reported case rates from 1966 to 1979. Major epidemics occurred every six to nine years, but in most communities the disease was endemic with a yearly occurrence peaking in spring (Fig. 9-2). In the United States, before the use of vaccine, 80% to 90% of the population had been infected by adulthood.

Rubella is such a benign illness that vaccine would not have been developed nor applied if prevention of child or adult illness were the aim. The impetus for vaccine development is to prevent congenital rubella. Intrauterine fetal infection may result in cardiac lesions, eye defects (particularly cataracts), deafness, growth retardation, thrombocytopenic purpura, hepatosplenomegaly, hepatitis, central nervous system (CNS) defects (psychomotor retardation, macrocephaly, encephalitis or asceptic meningitis), and lesions of the long bones. Late

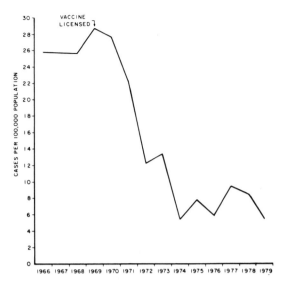

Fig. 9-1. Rubella (German measles): reported case rates by year, United States, 1966–1979. The reported incidence of rubella in 1979 was less than 20% of that reported in 1969, the year of vaccine licensure. (CDC, MMWR Annual Summary, 1979, 28:54, Sept 1980)

manifestations are diabetes mellitus, immunologic deficiency, and in rare cases, progressive panencephalitis. Multi-systemic involvement is common. With severely affected infants, the mortality is high—usually in infancy.

If rubella occurs in the first three months of pregnancy, the proportion of infants with defects at birth is approximately 16%. Because some defects such as deafness and psychomotor retardation become apparent later in childhood, the proportion with congenitally derived defects is actually 30% to 35%. The risk of defect is highest if the mother contracts rubella during the first month of pregnancy.

IMMUNIZING ANTIGEN

Rubella vaccine, a live attenuated virus vaccine, is now prepared in the United States solely in human diploid cells. Previous vaccines were prepared in duck embryo cell culture (HPVV-77) and in dog kidney cells (Cendehill). The virus has been attenuated by multiple passage in tissue culture (for example the current vaccine RA 27/3 was passaged 25 times in human diploid, W138 cells). All live rubella vaccines induce antibody response in at least 95% of recipients. They also result in recoverable virus in 75% of recipients, in lower titer than is found with natural rubella, and lasting for only one or two days. Numerous trials have shown that the virus is not communicable to others.

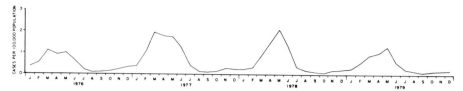

Fig. 9-2. Rubella (German measles): reported case rates by month, United States, 1976–1979. (CDC, MMWR Annual Summary, 1979, 28:54, Sept 1980)

The distinctive features of RA 27/3 (human diploid) vaccine are that it retains the ability to infect by a natural route (intranasally) and that it also produces a broader range of antibody responses than do the rubella vaccines that preceded it (HPV-77 and Cendehill). Another important feature is that it induces local secretory antibody in the oropharynx. It has been tested exhaustively for teratogenic potential (of particular concern because, in other respects, this strain retained some of the characteristics of natural rubella virus) and none has been found.

So far, the RA 27/3 vaccine has been extremely potent but has induced no excess of adverse reactions. A fourfold titer rise has been induced in virtually all vaccines. It is available alone, or in combination with measles vaccine (MR) or, additionally, with mumps vaccine (MMR). The triple vaccine (MMR) is recommended for routine infant-child vaccination.

IMMUNITY

Immunity to rubella appears to be a complex phenomenon. Both antibodies and cell-mediated immune (CMI) response are detectable after infection. Neutralizing antibody is protective against disease on reexposure but subclinical infection occurs in a few patients (4%). Recovery from primary infection may be unrelated to antibody synthesis or may be only partially dependent upon it. Cell-mediated immunity is probably important in recovery but its role in protection against reinfection is unclear.

Some insight is gained into rubella immunity through consideration of the experiences of those receiving passive antibodies during the incubation period of the disease. If enough antibodies are administered, infection develops but clinical disease is inapparent or mild. With larger amounts of antibodies, both infection and disease can be aborted, suggesting that neutralization of the virus by antibodies is an effective means of resisting infection.

Asymptomatic reinfection can occur after natural rubella; inapparent reinfection occurs more commonly in vaccinees. Of patients vaccinated with HPVV-77 or Cendehill, 50% to 80% were reinfected on exposure. Reinfection following vaccination with RA 27/3 vaccine appears to be much less frequent. Reinfection with viremia would be detrimental to the prevention of congenital rubella but reinfection without viremia might result in boosting immunity and adding to protective effect. In fact, reinfection does not cause detectable viremia or sufficient pharyngeal virus for transmission.

RATIONALE FOR IMMUNIZATION

There has been considerable debate about the optimal plan for rubella vaccination to prevent congenital rubella. The United States and the United Kingdom have chosen different strategies. In the U.S., the strategy has been to immunize preschool and elementary school children of both sexes, with the aim being the prevention of large-scale rubella epidemics, if not eradication of the disease itself. Such a strategy assumes long-lasting protection conferred by the vaccine, which appears to be true of both the HPV-77 vaccine and the currently used RA 27/3 preparation. Thus, pregnant women are protected by decreasing their exposure to the reservoir of epidemic rubella in their children. In contrast, the emphasis in the United Kingdom has been the vaccination of prepubertal girls alone.

In neither instance has the strategy been entirely successful. In a recent analysis, Knox used computer models to show that the current immunization rate in each country is inadequate and that it will lead to the accumulation of enough susceptible women of child-bearing age to result in a serious potential for congenital rubella. To date, the immunization program in the United Kingdom has been insufficient to yield a significant reduction in rubella among pregnant women and to decrease the incidence of congenital rubella. In the United Kingdom, although the rate of childhood rubella, and thus congenital rubella, has decreased considerably since the institution of the vaccination program, cases still occur, although there has been no major nationwide epidemic since 1964, and this decline is attributed to vaccine usage, incomplete as it is.

The major concern in the United States is that, despite the decreased incidence of rubella in children, the rate in those over 15 years of age has not diminished; the highest rates currently observed are in those 15 to 19 years old (Fig. 9-3). This is consistent with serologic studies that have shown persisting susceptibility of teenagers and young adults. In the pre-vaccine era, approximately 15% of postpubescent women were suscepti-

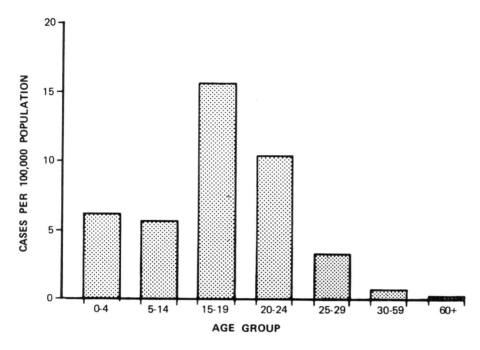

Fig. 9-3. Rubella (German measles): reported case rates by age group (excluding unknown ages), United States, 1979. (CDC, MMWR Annual Summary, 1979, 28:54, Sept 1980)

ble. Although nationwide surveys are not available, serologic surveys today show at least the same susceptibility pattern, and in some instances, as many as 23% of women are seronegative. Increased emphasis is needed in order to identify and immunize susceptible prepubertal adolescent girls and nonpregnant women.

Susceptible men and women who might expose pregnant women should be identified and immunized. It must be kept in mind that the most damaging exposure is in the first or second month of pregnancy, often before a woman is aware of her own pregnancy. In a number of recent episodes, rubella has been transmitted to pregnant women from infected health-care personnel, so that it is prudent to determine rubella susceptibility and to immunize susceptible physicians, nurses, and other members of the health profession in order to protect those patients.

Health care personnel are at particular risk when caring for infants with congenital rubella who may excrete the virus from several sites for months. It is thus particularly important to check the susceptibility of all who might be involved in such care and to restrict exposure to all but immune personnel.

SCHEDULING OF IMMUNIZATION

Rubella vaccination is recommended for all children, for many adolescents and for some adult patients, particularly nonpregnant female patients of child-bearing age. In infants, rubella immunization is recommended after 12 months of age so that persisting maternal immunity will not interfere with immunization. If the vaccination is given in combination with measles and mumps vaccine (MMR), which is the preferred method, then immunization should be delayed until 15 months as this is the optimal age for administration of live measles vaccine. In either instance, the vaccine is given in a single dose by the subcutaneous route. As no waning of immunity following vaccination has been documented, no further doses are necessary. Vaccination may be given at any age and should be given to all children and adult patients without histories of prior immunization or who are seronegative. There is no known adverse response to vaccination of immune individuals and serologic tests for antibody are not considered routinely necessary. However, the patient's history may be unreliable and serologic determination may be the only way to determine immunization status.

In vaccination of postpubertal girls and of women, care should be taken to assure that the recipient is not pregnant, as there are theoretic risks to such vaccination. This should be explained to the recipient, and pregnant women should be excluded. Since the great majority of women are immune, serologic testing for susceptibility can prevent unnecessary immunization if such testing is readily available.

SIDE-EFFECTS AND ADVERSE REACTIONS

Rash (10%) and lymphadenopathy (20%) may occur following vaccination. Fever (4%) is rare. Joint pain, particularly of the small joints, is not uncommon following vaccination although frank arthritis is rare. The frequency of arthralgia is dependent upon age, sex, and immunity. It does not occur in recipients with prior immunity and occurs most often in women (arthralgia has been reported in as many as 25% to 50% of female recipients). Arthralgia occurs in less than 10% of children and appears to be less frequent in RA 27/3 recipients. Although the pathogenesis of arthropathy following natural or vaccine rubella is not understood, vaccine virus has been recovered from effusions on a few occasions. Arthralgia usually occurs within one to three weeks after vaccination, although it has been reported as occurring as long as ten weeks later, and symptoms may recur over extended periods.

A rare complication of rubella vaccination is peripheral neuropathy. Paresthesias of the arm or hand, or bone pain and difficulty in extension, have been reported most often, primarily, with previous vaccine strains.

Rubella vaccine virus can frequently be recovered from the oropharynx of vaccine recipients. The virus is in lower titer and is present for a shorter duration than in natural rubella. There is no evidence that it is communicable, even though this has been extensively studied. Therefore, there is no contraindication to vaccination of the child of a pregnant woman. In fact, there is every reason to do so in order to protect the mother from the possibility of exposure to natural rubella in her child. It has been shown that if nursing mothers are vaccinated, vaccine virus may be excreted in their milk. This does not represent a contraindication to vaccination of the postpubertal mother, for, although transmission to the infant may occur, no untoward effect of such exposure has been documented.

CONTRAINDICATIONS

PREGNANCY

Rubella vaccine should not be given to pregnant women. Rubella vaccine virus can cross the placenta and infect the fetus. This has been well documented in approximately 25% of women who chose abortion. However, congenital malformations in the fetus exposed to vaccine virus have not been found. The Center for Disease Control (CDC) has well-documented data on 93 such instances. Three had evidence of fetal infection. Since the RA 27/3 strain of vaccine (human diploid) has been in use, there have been eight documented instances of inadvertent administration in susceptible pregnant women; all infants were carried to term and were healthy. Examination of the products of conception of 12 seronegative women vaccinated with this strain before abortion has failed to yield vaccine virus.

ALTERED IMMUNITY

Rubella vaccination (as is true for all live virus vaccines) is contraindicated in persons with altered immune status, including leukemia, lymphoma, or generalized malignancy, and in persons undergoing therapy with corticosteroids, alkylating drugs, antimetabolites, or radiation.

EPIDEMIC CONTROL

In the instance of a rubella outbreak, it is recommended that all persons without contraindications be vaccinated. There is no evidence that vaccination following exposure will prevent illness but there is no evidence that it is harmful to vaccinate someone who is incubating the disease. Rubella vaccine administered in the face of epidemic disease has been shown to become effective 14 to 21 days after immunization, suggesting that vaccination does not alter the course of disease in those incubating natural rubella virus but that if the vaccine virus is administered prior to exposure, infection is prevented.

Immune serum globulin (IG) given after rubella exposure will not prevent infection but may modify illness. The only indications for use might be following exposure of an individual with altered immune status or when rubella occurs in a pregnant woman who would not consider termination. In the latter instance, protection cannot be assured as infants with congenital rubella have been born to women given IG shortly after exposure (see Chapter 23). Counseling about fetal risk and the consequent management following exposure of a pregnant woman to rubella is difficult. Recent review of strategies behind such counseling and the suggestion of algorithm for their solution has been prepared by the CDC.

REFERENCES

Balfour HH, Groth KE, Edelman CK: RA 27/3 Rubella vaccine: A four-year followup. Am J Dis Child 134:350, 1980

Beasley RP: Dilemmas presented of the attenuated rubella vaccines. Am J Epidemiol 92:158, 1970

Center for Disease Control: Rubella surveillance—January 1976–December 1978. May, 1980

Fleet WF, Vaughn W, Lefkowitz LB et al: Gestational exposure to rubella vaccines. A population surveillance study. Am J Epidemiol 101:220, 1975

Hayden GF, Harrmann KL, Buimovici-Klein E et al: Subclinical congenital rubella infection associated with maternal rubella vaccination in early pregnancy. J Pediatr 96:869, 1980

Horstmann DM: Controlling rubella: Problems and perspectives. Ann Intern Med 83:412, 1975

Knox EG: Strategy for rubella vaccination. Int J Epidemiol 9:13, 1980

Krugman S (ed): Proceedings of the International Conference on Rubella Immunization. Am J Dis Child 118:3, 1969

Lerman SJ, Silver MR, Nankervis GA: Arthralgia and rubella immunization. Ann Intern Med 88:131, 1978

Preblud SR, Serdula MK, Frank JA et al: Rubella vaccination in the United States: A ten-year review. Epidemiol Rev 2:171, 1980

Schaffner W, Fleet WF, Kilroy AW et al: Polyneuropathy following rubella immunization: A followup study and a review of the problem. Am J Dis Child 127:684, 1974

Schoenbaum SC, Hyde JN, Bartoskesky L et al: Benefit-cost analysis of rubella vaccination policy. New Engl J Med 294:306, 1976

Weibel RE, Villarejos VM, Klein EB et al: Clinical and laboratory studies of live attenuated RA 27/3 and HPV 77-DE rubella virus vaccines. Proc Soc Exper Biol Med 165:44, 1980

Wyll SA, Hermann KL: Inadvertent rubella vaccination of pregnant women. JAMA 225:1472, 1978

10
Measles

Vincent A. Fulginiti

DISEASE

Today's practitioners see so little measles that many are unfamiliar with either the disease's manifestations or its ravages. This short synopsis should serve to remind us that the disease is worth preventing.

Measles (rubeola, hard measles, coughing measles, ten-day measles, morbilli, and red measles) is caused by a single type of paramyxovirus. The agent is an RNA virus with a lipid envelope from which hemagglutinin particles project. Although primates can be infected, humans are the only reservoir in nature.

After an incubation period of 8 to 13 days, a prodromal illness begins, consisting of high fever, conjunctivitis, coryza, and a harsh rasping cough. The prodrome usually lasts from 3 to 7 days; this is followed by the appearance of a generalized rash that begins on the face and hairline, lasts 4 to 7 days, and is generalized in a caudad fashion. The rash is maculopapular and erythematous and tends to be confluent. Just prior to its appearance or shortly thereafter, typical Koplik spots appear on the buccal mucosa and sometimes on the nasal mucosa. These characteristic tiny pinpoint white plaques on an erythematous base are pathognomonic of measles.

Uncomplicated measles may last for as long as two or three weeks although it is usually over within ten days. Uncomplicated measles is associated with moderate-to-severe disability, necessitating absence from school or from other activities during the symptomatic phase. Measles is contagious with a high degree of transmissibility, particularly during the prodromal period and within the first four days after the appearance of the rash. (See Figure 10-1 for reported case rates in the United States from 1950 to 1979.)

Measles tends to be more severe in infants, in those who are immunosuppressed, malnourished, or who have certain other diseases, and

113

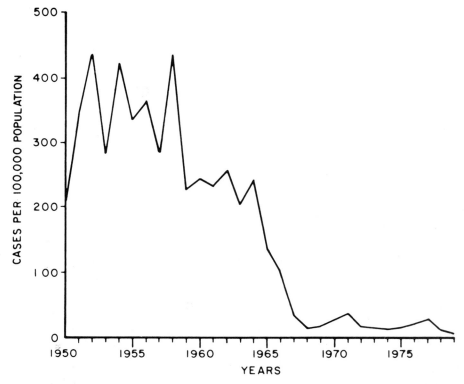

Fig. 10-1. Measles (rubeola): reported case rates by year, United States, 1950–1979. (CDC, MMWR Annual Summary, 1979, 28:54, Sept 1980)

in adult patients. Even without complications, measles in these categories of patients may be severe and even lethal.

Complications from measles include direct effects of the disease or bacterial superinfection. Measles pneumonia and encephalitis are the major complications of the virus infection. From 5% to 15% of patients experience bacterial superinfection including otitis media, sinusitis, pneumonia, and diarrhea. Hemorrhagic measles is a particularly severe form of the disease which is believed to be caused by disseminated intravascular coagulation.

A rare form of chronic measles infection develops in some children years after primary disease. Subacute sclerosing panencephalitis (SSPE) is an almost invariably lethal infection of the central nervous system (CNS) in which measles virus persists in an incomplete form in neurons of the CNS and causes symptoms years after primary infection which commonly occurs in infancy.

Atypical measles is a severe form of the disease that occurs in persons who received killed measles virus (KMV) vaccine. High fever, CNS symptoms, pneumonitis, polyserositis, pleural effusion, edema, and an atypical rash resembling that of Rocky Mountain Spotted fever all occur in such patients.

Since the advent of live measles virus (LMV) vaccine, the incidence of measles has decreased from more than 500,000 cases per year in 1962 to fewer than 15,000 reported in 1980. In addition, the epidemiology of the disease has altered dramatically in that older persons who escaped both measles immunization and the natural disease are now susceptible. Epidemics involving high-school-age, college-age, and young adult patients are common and although these outbreaks are occurring in fewer and fewer places, there is a considerable reservoir of unimmunized, uninfected persons and the potential for mini-epidemics persists. With an immunization rate of over 90% for school-age children in the U.S. in 1980, it is unlikely that we will experience much measles in this group. Depending upon the local immunization practices, school-age children and those not yet attending school may remain susceptible and experience the disease. Sometimes older adult patients also contract the disease; recently, a 33-year-old woman in California died from progressive measles. She was unimmunized and had previously escaped the disease.

In the United States at present, the goal is to eradicate measles by 1982 by offering immunization universally to infants at age 15 months and to seek all susceptible persons in the population and immunize them, regardless of age. Among those susceptible are the following:

Persons of any age who have not been immunized.

Persons who were immunized prior to 15 months of age. In this category are those who were immunized under 12 months of age; as many as 35% of such persons may be unprotected despite a history of receipt of vaccine. This phenomenon occurs because of persisting maternal antibody in sufficient quantity to inhibit immunization. Few children between the ages of 12 and 15 months escape immunization but according to some studies, as many as 15% immunized at age 12 or 13 months may remain susceptible.

Primary vaccine failures. Regardless of the age of immunization after 15 months of age, LMV vaccine will only protect from 95% to 98% of recipients. Thus, a few persons remain susceptible despite vaccination.

True vaccine failures. There are few if any reports of persons adequately immunized as demonstrated by antibody elevation following immunization who remain susceptible. Thus, true vaccine failures probably do not occur or occur at such an extremely low frequency as to be discounted.

Recipients of KMV vaccine. Prior to 1968, KMV vaccine was available and widely used; as many as 800,000 individuals in the U.S. and many thousands more in Canada (through 1970) received this vaccine. As will be detailed later, KMV vaccine did not immunize these recipients because they retain a lifelong susceptibility to atypical measles upon exposure to the natural disease.

Improper administration of vaccine. When measles vaccine was first introduced, it was prepared in liquid form and it has undergone several manufacturing changes since then. As a result, some persons who were immunized received an impotent product because of mishandling prior to administration. For example, freezing was necessary for the liquid form of vaccine and, on occasion, the liquid warmed, which destroyed the virus. The use of immune serum globulin along with measles vaccine resulted in some mishaps. Some physicians inadvertently mixed the two products together or administered them at the same site simultaneously. The measles antibody in the immune serum globulin combined with the measles virus in the vaccine, inactivating it, and leaving the recipient susceptible.

It is unknown what proportion of former vaccine recipients are nonimmune because of such mechanical failures. Short of specific antibody testing, there is no way to be certain of a patient's status within this group.

Thus, a large group of persons in today's population are immune as a result of contracting the natural infection before the introduction of measles vaccine in 1961. After 1961, the population can be broken down into various subgroups: those who are immune by virtue of immunization; those who are immune as a result of contracting the natural disease; and those who are susceptible because of lack of immunization or improperly received immunization, or for any of the reasons cited above.

IMMUNIZING ANTIGEN

KILLED MEASLES VIRUS VACCINE

Although no longer available or used, KMV vaccine was given to more than 800,000 persons in the United States prior to 1968 and in Canada prior to 1970. KMV vaccine was prepared by inactivating live virus grown in tissues derived from monkeys or from hens' eggs. Adjuvant was added to the final formulation and it was administered alone or prior to LMV vaccine. The usual series consisted of two or three doses of KMV with subsequent booster doses of KMV or a dose of LMV.

Inactivated vaccine resulted in antibody production in recipients with short-lived immunity. After a varying period, usually six months or longer, recipients of KMV became susceptible to atypical reactions to either attenuated or wild virus. Administration of LMV was associated with local reactions (heat, induration, and pain and rash at the site of inoculation) and occasionally with systemic reactions (fever, regional adenopathy, headache, and malaise). Exposure to wild virus could result in a bizarre disease with an atypical eruption (atypical distribution with peripheral accentuation and onset of rash, vesicles, petechia, and purpura), severe systemic symptoms (fever, headache, lethergy, and uncoordination), and specific tissue symptoms (pneumonia, polyserositis, and pleural and peritoneal signs and symptoms). Extremely high antibody titers and a skin reaction thought to be of the delayed hypersensitivity type were noted.

LIVE MEASLES VIRUS VACCINE

Two major types of LMV have been developed. The original LMV was derived from the Edmonston strain of measles virus isolated by Enders and colleagues. An attenuated virus was obtained after many passages in chick embryo tissue culture. This agent (Edmonston B) produced minimal symptoms and reliable immunity. However, the 15% incidence of rash and the 80% incidence of fever were judged too severe to allow routine use of this product. Simultaneous but separate administration of measles immune globulin (MIG) reduced the incidence of fever and rash to more acceptable levels without significantly sacrificing immunity.

A second source of attenuated virus was developed by Schwarz by additional passage in chick embryo tissue culture. This further attenuated measles virus (FAMV) produced fewer febrile or exanthematous reactions but resulted in lower levels of antibody that decreased more rapidly and to a greater degree than did the antibody induced by Edmonston B immunization. Despite this decline, recipients appeared to be equally protected against natural exposure in subsequent years. The FAMV vaccine does not necessitate the simultaneous administration of MIG.

Initially, LMV was prepared in either chick embryo tissue culture or canine kidney tissue culture. Today, only a single FAMV product is available in the United States, and it is prepared in chick embryo tissue culture. No other form of LMV is currently available to the practicing physician in the United States. The LMV is supplied in lyophilized form for reconstitution just prior to immunization, thus avoiding many of the potency-reducing factors previously discussed. The manufacturer's directions should be followed explicitly in the storage, reconstitution, and administration of LMV. The virus is fragile and may be rendered inactive if any of these steps is omitted or changed significantly. Heating the vaccine, adding the improper diluent, using glass syringes, or mixing with immune globulin can result in inactivation of the virus and failure to immunize a susceptible patient.

It is no longer advisable or necessary to use immune serum globulin of any type in conjunction with LMV vaccine.

RATIONALE FOR ACTIVE IMMUNIZATION AGAINST MEASLES

Protection against measles is desirable because of the morbidity and occasional mortality associated with the natural disease (Fig. 10-2). As was indicated, measles produces disability sufficient to result in absence from school or from other activities, and a significant number of those infected experience severe and even life-threatening complications.

In the past, measles in the first year of life occurred with sufficient frequency that it was desirable to offer protection as early as was feasible. The recommendation when LMV was first introduced was to immunize at 9 months of age. This age was selected because it was believed that maternally transmitted transplacental antibody had waned sufficiently by that age to permit immunization. Subsequent experience indicated that as many as 35% of recipients at 9 months of age failed to become immunized because of the presence of maternally derived neutralizing antibody. As a result, the recommendation was changed and LMV vaccine was offered to patients at 12 months of age. In recent years, we have had conflicting reports concerning the adequacy of immunization at 12 and 13 months of age. Results of four separate studies indicated that as many as 15% of vaccinees at 12 or 13 months of age were not immunized, again believed to be secondary to small amounts of persisting maternal antibody. Thus, a national recommendation was made to begin immunization at 15 months of age, and this recommendation still stands. However, in the intervening years, several additional studies have been performed which suggest that, at least in some population groups, adequate immunization can be achieved at 12 months and waiting until 15 months does not enhance the immunization rate. Despite this conflicting evidence, the advisory bodies are still recommending that children be immunized at 15 months of age.

A special situation pertains if measles is endemic, and those who are likely to come in contact with cases of measles are immunized at any age from 6 months onward. If a child must be immunized before he is 15 months old then a second dose of LMV vaccine should be administered once the child is 15 months old. From consideration of the immunology

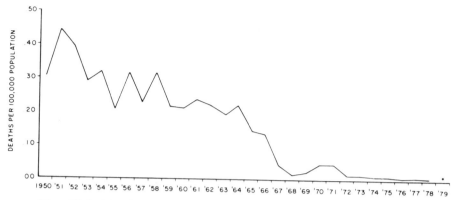

Fig. 10-2. Measles (rubeola): reported death rates by year, United States, 1950–1978. (CDC, MMWR Annual Summary, 1979, 28:54, Sept 1980)

involved, one should recognize that a certain proportion of those immunized prior to 15 months of age will have had successful immunization. Limited data indicate that receipt of the second LMV vaccine should produce no untoward reactions. On the other hand, those who escape immunization despite administration of LMV prior to 15 months of age may be successfully immunized once they attain the age of 15 months. Even here there is conflicting evidence. The results of a study conducted by Jeanette Wilkins suggest that those immunized early in life, when reimmunized after 15 months of age, may have only a transient antibody response which diminishes with time. She suggests that such individuals may remain immune despite receipt of the two doses of LMV. This issue was unresolved as this chapter was written, because only 38 infants were included in her initial study, and only a small portion of these exhibited this phenomenon. To our knowledge, the study has not been duplicated and administration of the second dose of LMV vaccine to those immunized prior to 15 months of age is recommended.

Measles vaccine may be administered at any age to a nonimmune susceptible person. If one immunizes an adolescent or adult patient, one can expect a greater reaction rate of systemic subjective symtomatology. Such a patient will more often complain of headache, lassitude, anorexia, and the like than will an infant or a young child.

IMMUNITY AGAINST MEASLES

It appears clear that recovery from measles virus infection is not antibody-dependent. Rather, an intact lymphocyte-mediated cell-mediated immune (CMI) response is responsible for limiting the spread of measles virus and for terminating an acute infection. Experience among persons who are incapable of mounting antibody responses, such as those with B-cell immunodeficiencies, has provided evidence for this relationship. In such patients, natural measles infection undergoes a normal course despite the lack of antibody. It is believed that such patients recover because their CMI responses are intact and are thus capable of limiting and eliminating measles virus. Conversely, those with T-cell deficiencies who cannot mount sufficient CMI responses to measles virus will experience extensive and often lethal infection.

On the other hand, antibodies appear to play a major role in protection against reinfection. Those who have detectable measles-neutralizing antibody activity in their serum will not develop the disease despite intensive exposure. It is believed that circulating measles antibody is sufficient to neutralize measles virus introduced into the respiratory tract. In addition, such persons have also demonstrable local IgA antibodies which also play a role in neutralizing the virus and in preventing systemic infection, and persistent CMI may play a role.

Those who have received KMV vaccine have altered immunologic reactivity to measles virus. There are two major theories to account for this altered reactivity. First, I believe that CMI responses are accentuated in such patients. When the original antibody stimulated by KMV is lost, the CMI hyperreactivity results in extreme sensitivity to measles virus and the atypical measles syndrome. However, Bellanti and associates believe that an Arthus reaction is responsible for the altered reactivity. They believe that preformed antibody as a result of KMV is present in the serum but not in the respiratory secretions; for example, there is no topical IgA antibody present. As a result, when virus is introduced into the respiratory tract, it multiplies unmolested, stimulating further production of serum antibody which produces an antigen-antibody complex that is responsible for both the local skin manifestations and the systemic signs and symptoms of the disease. At this point, the issue is unresolved and there is evidence for both theses.

One peculiar aspect of measles immunology is the occurrence of SSPE. In such patients, the measles virus appears to gain access to CNS neurons and to remain inactive there in incomplete form. That is, the virus does not develop its usual capsid and envelope structure but remains within the cell as an active genome. At some point, multiplication is sufficient to cause the degenerative CNS infection known as SSPE. Antibodies appear to be produced locally as a result of the persistent measles virus infection and can be detected in the spinal fluid of such individuals. During the clinical manifestations of SSPE, very high, often phenomenal, levels of serum antibody can be detected. The immunology of SSPE is not completely understood and we do not have an adequate explanation either for the persistence of the virus in the neuron or for its emergence to produce clinical disease. Many of those with SSPE were infected very early in life. It is possible that circulating antibodies produce an active-passive infectious experience in which the virus is confined to the neuron because of circulating antibodies, enabling it to persist there in incomplete form.

Finally, anyone with detectable circulating antibodies at the time of measles exposure is believed to be immune to measles. There has been no documented second case of measles in a person with either naturally acquired antibodies or antibodies acquired after LMV immunization.

SCHEDULING OF MEASLES IMMUNIZATION

Certain precautions are advisable in LMV use. First, whenever feasible, a negative tuberculin test should be obtained prior to LMV administration. This precaution is less important today than when the vaccine was first introduced. The rationale behind it was that natural measles was known to exacerbate silent or minimally symptomatic tuberculosis and it was feared that the vaccine infection might do the same. Such fears have not been realized and the Public Health Service has abandoned this particular precaution. In individual practice, however, the Academy of Pediatrics still recommends that tuberculin screening be done simultaneously with or prior to LMV immunization. In usual practice, this means that a child would undergo a tuberculin test at 12 months of age and LMV vaccination at 15 months of age.

Second, febrile illnesses usually contraindicate LMV administration. Only healthy children should receive any live virus vaccine.

Third, any defect in CMI is a contraindication to LMV administration; it is also prudent to avoid LMV in any child with congenital or acquired immunodeficiency.

Fourth, LMV should not be given for two to three months following immune serum globulin administration. Measles-neutralizing antibodies in immune globulin can counteract effective immunization.

Last, pregnancy is a contraindication for LMV use. This is a theoretic risk and no adverse consequences have been associated with LMV use in pregnancy. However, no live virus vaccine should be injected during gestation for fear of potential harm to the fetus.

In the past, LMV use was thought to be contraindicated in egg-sensitive persons. Considerable experience has shown that the chick embryo vaccine in which LMV is prepared does not contain egg antigens. *Its use in children who are egg-sensitive is not contraindicated.*

PRIMARY IMMUNIZATION WITH LIVE MEASLES VIRUS

The usual dose of currently available FAMV is 0.5 ml given subcutaneously. Live measles virus vaccine should be administered routinely at 15 months of age or any age thereafter. In normal well-child practice, LMV should be administered to all infants when they achieve this age. It is unnecessary to use IG in any form or amount concomitant with the currently available LMV.

IMMUNIZATION OF CHILDREN PREVIOUSLY IMMUNIZED WITH KILLED MEASLES VIRUS

Because children previously immunized with KMV may experience untoward reactions to LMV and are susceptible to atypical measles on exposure to wild virus, specific discussion with parents and consent for further use of measles vaccine should be obtained.

The recommendation is that such children be immunized with single subcutaneous doses of LMV at any interval after receipt of KMV vaccine. In 10% to 50% of children, one can expect local reactions consisting of heat, induration, and tenderness. In 3% to 10% of children, systemic symptoms such as fever, malaise, and regional adenopathy may occur. I have encountered reactions severe enough to necessitate hospitalization. Although experimental evidence suggests that 0.1 ml of LMV administered intradermally reduces local and systemic reactions and still results in adequate antibody stimulation, this cannot be considered a routine or recommended practice.

COMBINATION OF LIVE VIRUS VACCINES

Live measles virus vaccine is most often administered in combination with rubella and mumps virus vaccines (MMR). It also may be administered separately or in combination with rubella virus vaccine (see Chapter 23).

SPECIAL CIRCUMSTANCES

If an unimmunized child is exposed to natural measles and promptly brought to a physician's attention, LMV administration may result in prevention of measles. This protection occurs because LMV has a shorter incubation period than does natural measles (7 days as opposed to 11 days). The LMV should be administered as soon after exposure as is possible, certainly within the first 48 to 72 hours.

If clinical tuberculosis is present or if the unimmunized child has a positive tuberculin test, measles prevention is desirable. If the clinical tuberculosis is under adequate chemotherapy, LMV can be administered. In a child with a newly discovered positive tuberculin test, it is advisable to administer INH for at least two weeks prior to receipt of LMV. Temporary depression of tuberculin sensitivity may occur following LMV administration, commencing 4 to 7 days and lasting several weeks.

Children who have received their original LMV prior to 12 months of age should be given second doses of LMV at any age, because protection from the first dose is uncertain.

In measles epidemics with high risk of exposure in infants, one may wish to immunize infants between 6 and 15 months of age with LMV. It must be appreciated that some infants will not be immunized but will be protected by natural transplacental immunity. All infants immunized in this fashion during epidemic conditions who are under 15 months of age must receive second doses of LMV at or after 15 months of age (see previous discussion).

For those who cannot be given LMV because of risks associated with underlying disease conditions or age, one must consider use of preventive amounts of IG on exposure.

RECALL IMMUNIZATION

Those who have received LMV vaccine at or after 15 months of age do not need any further doses of this vaccine. Some experts are advising universal reimmunization for all children irrespective of history. I and various recommending bodies have not adopted this policy. Theoretic risks, the fact that at least 90% of persons are already immune, and diversion of limited resources recommend that universal reimmunization not be undertaken.

SIDE-EFFECTS OF MEASLES IMMUNIZATION

With the current vaccine, no more than 15% of children should experience fever and rash 5 to 12 days after receipt of LMV. These reactions may be clinically inapparent or may result in mild disability.

No other side-effects have been observed with LMV administration.

Those who have received KMV vaccine in the past may experience local reactions as previously discussed.

ADVERSE REACTIONS ATTRIBUTABLE TO LIVE MEASLES VIRUS VACCINE

Live measles virus vaccination has resulted in disseminated disease and death in those with depressed immune function involving absent or diminished CMI. Children with congenital T-cell deficiencies or acquired CMI deficiencies secondary to such diseases as leukemia and lymphoma or secondary to the administration of potent chemotherapeutic agents are potentially susceptible to this complication.

Although a variety of acute CNS disorders have occurred within 30 days of LMV administration, none has definitely been attributed to LMV and a few have been identified as caused by other viruses. In the aggregate, LMV prevents more encephalitis by preventing natural measles than it can possibly induce.

Some feel that SSPE may be the result of LMV administration. However, this relationship is speculative and uncertain because a long interval elapses between the original natural measles virus infection and the manifestations of SSPE. Many of these children may have had mild or inapparent natural measles infection prior to receipt of LMV. Thus, it is uncertain whether any cases of SSPE can be directly attributable to LMV vaccine.

Theoretically, tuberculosis can be exacerbated by LMV administration. Several instances of tuberculous meningitis were described within 30 days of LMV administration during the initial measles campaigns. However, there has been no direct evidence of worsening tuberculosis or of tuberculosis secondary to LMV. Treated tuberculosis is not a contraindication to measles vaccine.

SPECIFIC PRECAUTIONS

As was already noted, LMV should not be administered to anyone who is immunosuppressed either by congenital or acquired disease or treatment, partcularly those that suppress CMI function. Live measles vaccine should not be administered knowingly to anyone with active clinical tuberculosis or a positive tuberculin test, unless such a person is treated.

Pregnancy is an absolute contraindication to LMV administration, although the risk is totally theoretic at present. Previous recipients of KMV vaccine may experience significant local and systemic reactions, as described previously. Live measles vaccine is not contraindicated for children who are egg-sensitive because the vaccine is prepared in chick embryo culture and does not contain egg antigens.

PASSIVE IMMUNIZATION

Immune globulin contains a variable amount of measles antibody; a formerly available product, measles immune globulin is no longer distributed. This product contained measured amounts of measles antibody. Immune globulin may be used to prevent or modify measles in an exposed, susceptible patient. I believe that prevention of measles with subsequent LMV immunization should be the goal of IG use. To accomplish this, 0.25 ml/kg of IG is administered within 6 days of exposure, and LMV administered 3 months later (see Chapter 23).

REFERENCES

Albrecht P, Ennis FA, Staltzman EJ et al: Persistence of maternal antibody in infants beyond 12 months of age: Mechanisms of measles vaccine failure. J Pediatr 91:715, 1977

Berman PH, Giles JP, Krugman S: Correlation of measles and subacute sclerosing panencephalitis. Neurology 18:91, 1968

Cherry JD: The new epidemiology of measles and rubella. Hosp Pract 15(7):49–57, 1980

Enders JF, Katz SL, Milanovic MJ et al: Studies on an attenuated measles virus vaccine. New Engl J Med 263:153–156, 1960

Fulginiti VA: Simultaneous measles exposure and immunization. Arch Gesamte Virusforsch 16:300–304, 1964

Fulginiti VA, Arthur JH: Altered reactivity to measles virus: Skin test reactivity and antibody response to measles virus antigens in recipients of killed measles virus vaccines. J Pediatr 75:609, 616, 1969

Fulginiti VA, Arthur JH, Pearlman DJ et al: Altered reactivity to measles virus: Local reactions following attenuated measles virus immunization in children who previously received a combination of inactivated and attenuated vaccines. Am J Dis Child 115:671–676, 1968

Fulginiti VA, Eller JJ, Downie AW et al: Altered reactivity to measles virus: Atypical measles in children previously immunized with inactivated measles vaccine. JAMA 202:1075–1077, 1967

Fulginiti VA, Helfer RE: Atypical measles in adolescent siblings 16 years after killed measles virus vaccine. JAMA 244:804–806, 1980

Fulginiti VA, Kempe CH: Measles exposure among vaccine recipients. Am J Dis Child 106:450–461, 1963

Hall WJ, Hall CB: Atypical measles in adolescents. Ann Intern Med 90:882–886, 1979

Hinman AR, Brandling-Bennett AD, Bernier RH et al: Current features of measles in the United States: Feasibility of measles elimination. Epidemiol Rev 2:153–170, 1980

Kempe CH, Fulginiti VA: The pathogenesis of measles. Arch Gesamte Virusforsch 16:103–128, 1964

Krause PJ, Cherry JD, Deseda-Tous J et al: Epidemic measles in young adults. Ann Intern Med 90:873–876, 1979

Krause PJ, Cherry JD, Naiditch MJ et al: Revaccination of previous recipients of killed measles vaccine: Clinical and immunologic studies. J Pediatr 93:565–571, 1978

Krugman RD, Rosenberg R, McIntosh K et al: Impotency of live-virus vaccines as a result of improper handling in clinical practice. J Pediatr 85:512–514, 1974

Krugman S: Present status of measles and rubella immunizations in the United States: A medical progress report. J Pediatr 90:1–5, 1977

Schwarz AJF: Preliminary tests of a highly attenuated measles vaccine. Am J Dis Child 103:386:389 1962

11
Mumps

James F. Jones

DISEASE

Mumps virus infection usually causes febrile parotitis. However, 30% to 40% of infections are asymptomatic. In the prevaccine era, more than 90% of susceptible persons were infected by 15 years of age.

Mumps virus infection is not limited to the salivary glands. Twenty-five percent of those affected may have symptoms of aseptic meningitis, orchitis, or oophoritis. Frequently (30%–40%), those with meningitis do not have parotitis. Uncommon associations with mumps virus include encephalitis, transverse myelitis, unilateral deafness, Guillain-Barre syndrome, myocarditis, hepatitis, polyarteritis, thyroiditis, and nephritis. Recently, this virus has been incriminated in lower respiratory tract infections and in diabetes mellitus secondary to pancreatitis.

The disease occurs throughout the world and humans appear to be the only reservoir. Children are most susceptible; boys from 2 to 6 years of age have the highest infection rate. The virus is spread via salivary secretions for six days prior to clinical parotitis, and then continues to be shed for another 7 to 14 days. Urinary excretion may also persist for 2 to 3 weeks after clinical symptoms begin. The patient is contagious for a total of 4 weeks.

IMMUNIZING ANTIGEN

The virus used to prepare the vaccine currently available in the United States was first isolated from a patient with unilateral parotitis in 1963 by passage in embryonated hens' eggs. The virus was attenuated by 17 passages in primary chick embryo cell cultures before clarification (removal of cellular debris) and use as a vaccine (LMuV). The material is devoid of chicken antigens. The reconstituted vaccine also contains 25 μg of neomycin.

Formalin-killed mumps vaccines have not been available in the United States since 1969. Those who received this vaccine are considered nonimmune.

RATIONALE FOR ACTIVE IMMUNIZATION AGAINST MUMPS

Prevention of mumps is predicated upon substitution of attenuated virus infection for the natural disease. The early history of mumps immunization included use of a killed virus vaccine, which offered little protection for a short period. But when LMuV, was developed, there was considerable controversy about its use.

After LMuV was licensed, it was recommended for the selective immunization of susceptible children approaching puberty and of adult patients, particularly men with no history of mumps. This recommendation for selective use resulted from a lack of information about the vaccine's effectiveness and safety. As late as 1977, the British questioned the usefulness of the vaccine in anyone other than those mentioned above. They cited the low incidence of serious problems from the disease and the uncertain economic cost-to-benefit ratio of wider application of the vaccine.

With continued use and evaluation of the vaccine, the initial recommendation has been amended. The children who were originally immunized in 1965 have been observed for periods of up to 141 months. Mean serum antibody titers in these children fell only 27% over this time, compared with an 80% decrease in the antibody levels in control children after natural infection. The geometric mean titers in each group were comparable after this interval: 9.5 for the immunized group and 11.5 for the naturally infected group.

The decrease in the reported cases of the disease is another cited measurement of the effectiveness of the attenuated live vaccine (Fig. 11-1). In the United States, the number of reported cases has decreased from 200,000 per year before 1967 to approximately 20,000 per year in 1977. In areas such as Massachusetts, where a concerted effort has been made to immunize the population, the number of reported cases has decreased from approximately 12,000 to 100 per year. Estimated savings in Massachusetts by mumps prevention have been approximately $900,000. Similar savings have been calculated in other states and countries.

Because humans are the only known carriers of the disease, and immunization rates approaching 90% of children under 2 years of age have been obtained in such areas as King's County, Washington, the possibility of eradicating the disease has been predicted.

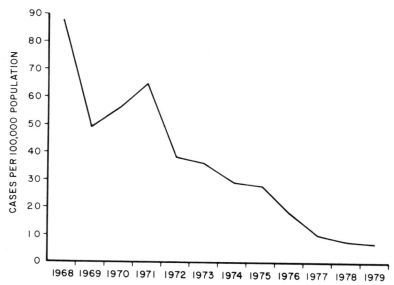

Fig. 11-1. Mumps: reported case rates by year, United States, 1968– 1979. In 1979, the reported incidence of mumps reached its lowest level since mumps became nationally notifiable in 1968. (CDC, MMWR Annual Summary, 1979, 28:54, Sept 1980)

IMMUNITY

Recovery from mumps infection is associated with production of antibody against the virus nucleocapsid (*S* or soluble antigen) and the surface hemagglutinin (V antigen), and with development of cell-mediated immunity (CMI). Complement-fixing (CF) antibodies to the S antigen peak within a week of onset and decline to undetectable levels over the following 6 to 12 months. The anti-V antibody peak usually doesn't occur until 2 to 3 weeks and then persists indefinitely. Cell-mediated immunity is detectable within 3 weeks of infection and persists indefinitely. The precise role of these specific immune parameters and the role of nonspecific factors in the resolution of mumps are unknown.

Protection against infection is most closely associated with persistence of adequate serum levels of anti-V antibody, although levels of this antibody as quantitated by CF testing may fall to undetectable levels. Neutralizing antibody levels have been suggested as the most reliable index of immunity. However, several persons have been identified who had no neutralizing antibodies but had positive evidence of CMI to mumps virus. When challenged with live vaccine, they did not produce neutralizing antibody and had various changes in their CMI responses on postimmunization specimens. These observations support the concept that CMI responses are also important in protection against infection.

Mumps virus antigens cross-react significantly with similar antigens of other paramyxoviruses, such as parainfluenza viruses. This phenomenon complicates both the interpretation of mumps serology and the determination of specific roles of antibody and CMI in mumps immunity. This issue is still unresolved.

Mumps vaccine induces an array of antibody and CMI responses, but which of these correlates with protection is uncertain.

SCHEDULING OF IMMUNIZATION

Mumps vaccine is now recommended for routine administration in infancy, usually in combination with measles and rubella virus vaccines at age 15 months. It may be given alone after 12 months of age; whether maternal antibody adversely affects the infant's response, as in measles, is not known. If monovalent mumps vaccine is given prior to age 15 months, some experts recommend using trivalent MMR (measles, mumps, rubella vaccines) at 15 months of age. The vaccine appears to be effective and protection lasts at least 12 years.

If for any reason mumps vaccine is not administered in infancy, it can be given at any age after 12 months. Parents, especially fathers, may not have a history of mumps infection in childhood, and it is desirable to immunize all with negative histories despite the fact that 30% to 40% of mumps infection is asymptomatic and the vaccine is unnecessary in some of these parents. There is no certain economical or feasible way to determine mumps immunity.

As with other live vaccines, no booster dose is needed. Post exposure administration of LMuV has not been shown to be effective, but is not contraindicated. Some physicians may elect to administer LMuV to men exposed to mumps. Such administration will not prevent mumps from the current exposure, but if mumps is not experienced, may confer immunity against further exposures.

Mumps can be disruptive in institutional settings. On entry, all prospective residents should be given mumps vaccine unless there is unequivocable evidence of past infection or immunization.

SIDE-EFFECTS

Reactions to LMuV have been few but include parotitis and fever. One case of orchitis has been reported in Europe. Other self-limited reactions including rash, pruritis, and purpura have also been reported.

Central nervous system (CNS) illness within 2 months of immunization has occurred following 22 of 32 million doses given. Mumps could not be proved as the cause of these illnesses. The incidence of vaccine-attributable CNS illness can be estimated at 0.9 instances per million doses distributed, which is much lower than the encephalitis rate of 2,600 per million cases. The vaccine-associated CNS problems are still less than 2.5 per million, if they occur at all.

Mumps virus crosses the placenta and, although no fetal infections have been recorded, LMuV is not recommended for pregnant women.

PASSIVE IMMUNIZATION

Immune globulin is not recommended for routine use in the prophylaxis or treatment of mumps. Mumps immune globulin is no longer available.

REFERENCES

Bader M: Mumps in Seattle-King County, Washington, 1920–1976. Am J Pub Health 67:1089–1091, 1977

Biedel CW: Recurrent mumps parotitis following natural infection and immunization. Am J Dis Child 132:678–680, 1978

Black FL, Houghton WJ: The significance of mumps hemagglutination inhibition titers in normal populations. Am J Epidemiol 85:101–107, 1967

Chiba Y, Dzierba JC, Morag AS et al: Cell-mediated immune response to mumps virus infection in man. J Immunol 116:12, 1976

Freeman R, Hambling MH: Serological studies on 40 cases of mumps virus infection. J Clin Pathol 33:28–32, 1980

Hayden GF, Preblud SR, Orenstein WA et al: Current status of mumps and mumps vaccine in the United States. Pediatrics 62:965–969, 1978

Jones JF, Ray CG, Fulginiti VA: Perinatal mumps infection. J Pediatr 96:912–914, 1980

Levitt LP, Mahoney DH, Casey HL et al: Mumps in a general population. Am J Dis Child 120:134–138, 1970

Lewis JE, Chernesky MA, Rawls ML et al: Epidemic of mumps in a partially immune population. CMA Journal 121:751–754, 1979

Mortimer PP: Mumps prophylaxis in the light of a new test for antibody. Br Med J 2:1523–1524, 1978

St. Geme JW, Yamauchi T, Eisenkalm EJ et al: Immunologic significance of the mumps virus skin test in infants, children and adults. Am J Epidemiol 101:253–263, 1975

Tsutsumi H, Chiba Y, Wataru A et al: T-cell-mediated cytotoxic response to mumps in humans. Infect Immunol 30:129–134, 1980

Weibel RE, Buynak E, McLean AA et al: Followup surveillance in human subjects following live attenuated measles, mumps and rubella virus vaccines. Proc Soc Exper Biol Med 162:328–332, 1979

Wilkins J, Williams FF, Wehrle PF: Infants' responses to live, attenuated, B level, Jeryl Lynn mumps vaccine. Am J Dis Child 124:66–67, 1972

Young NA: Chickenpox, measles and mumps. In: Remington JS, Klein JO (eds), Infectious Diseases of the Fetus and Newborn Infant, pp 521–586. Philadelphia, WB Saunders, 1976

12
Poliomyelitis

C. George Ray

DISEASE

Although poliomyelitis has probably been an infectious problem since antiquity, it was not widely recognized until the late 19th century, when severe outbreaks were first described in Europe and later in the United States.

The serotypes of poliovirus, types 1, 2 and 3, all produce similar spectra of clinical manifestations ranging from asymptomatic infection to overt paralytic disease. The hallmark of paralytic poliomyelitis, which develops in an estimated 1% to 2% of all infections, is asymmetric, flaccid paralysis of the extremities, with or without bulbar palsies. These features are almost unique for poliovirus infections; however, other enterovirus infections—notably Coxsackievirus A7 and enterovirus 71—have been regarded as important causes of this syndrome, particularly in Eastern Europe.

The transmission is primarily by fecal-oral routes in suboptimal hygienic settings, but aerosol or contact spread through oropharyngeal virus shedding can also occur. Since the widespread use of poliovirus vaccines began in 1955, there has been a dramatic reduction in paralytic cases in the United States (Figs. 12-1 and 12-2). Currently, the major portion of such cases are either imported (especially type 1 infections from Mexico) or are associated with live virus vaccine. However, the viruses are still widespread, particularly in underdeveloped countries, and the nearly total disappearance of wild polioviruses in the United States should not be interpreted as reassuring. Recent experience in developing countries has amply demonstrated how readily the viruses can be reintroduced into nonimmunized groups, with resultant severe outbreaks of disease. In 1978, the United States Immunization Survey found that only 60% of 1- to 4-year-old children had completed a full

133

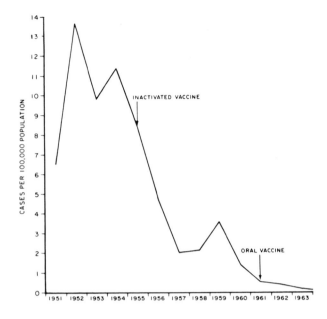

Fig. 12-1. Poliomyelitis (paralytic): reported case rates by year, United States, 1951–1963. (CDC, MMWR Annual Summary, 1979, 28:54, Sept 1980)

primary immunization series with poliovirus vaccine. This figure has presumably improved since then; however, there is still considerable concern about the large number of children and adults who remain susceptible and about the fact that such persons are often clustered together in contact groups that could facilitate rapid spread of infection by a wild virus.

IMMUNIZING ANTIGENS

Two types of poliovirus vaccines are currently licensed in the U.S. Which is the most desirable for routine use was extensively debated in the early 1960s and this discussion has been recently reopened (see references by Salk, Melnick, and Fox). In this chapter, we will outline the current recommendations for each vaccine, recognizing as objectively as possible the arguments in support of each. The reader clearly has some options in choosing which preparation is preferable in different situations and those decisions should be made on the basis of the data provided. One significant limitation faced by Public Health authorities is that inactivated poliovirus (IPV) vaccine is much more difficult to produce in a large supply than is the live, attenuated type, and this production problem is expected to continue.

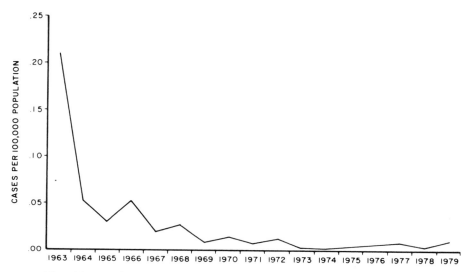

Fig. 12-2. Poliomyelitis (paralytic): reported case rates by year, United States, 1963–1979. (CDC, MMWR Annual Summary, 1979, 28:54, Sept 1980)

INACTIVATED POLIOVIRUS VACCINE

Inactivated polio vaccine (also referred to as killed polio vaccine, or Salk vaccine) was first licensed in 1955 and its use has been associated with a dramatic decline in the number of paralytic cases. It is still the only vaccine used in some countries, notably Sweden, Finland, and the Netherlands, and has proven highly effective. After 1962, IPV was largely replaced by oral polio vaccine in the United States, and only recently has IPV again become readily available. (Under investigation at present are several very potent IPV preparations manufactured in Germany and France. Antigenic and safety tests are being conducted in children under auspices of the Center for Disease Control [CDC].) The current vaccine, produced by Connaught Laboratories in Canada, is antigenically more potent than the original product, and can be obtained from Elkins-Sinn, Inc., 2 Esterbrook Lane, Cherry Hill, New Jersey, 08802.

The vaccine is given by means of subcutaneous injection. Primary vaccination with four doses of IPV produces antibody response to all three poliovirus serotypes in more than 95% of recipients; however, long-term experience with the more potent IPV now in use has not been sufficient to establish duration of immunity. Booster recommendations are based on observations from other countries where IPV has been in use for a longer time.

While IPV clearly diminishes the circulation of wild poliovirus strains, IPV recipients can be infected with either wild or attenuated live poliovirus strains, with resultant transient intestinal carriage. Nevertheless, the risk of such infection and carriage is diminished as compared with that of nonimmune persons, and if this occurs, the deleterious effects on the IPV-immunized individual are nil. The argument about whether such intestinal carriage poses a risk to nonimmune contacts continues.

Untoward paralytic complications have not been a problem in IPV recipients since the unfortunate 1955 "Cutter incident". In that episode, a cluster of poliomyelitis cases was related to vaccine that had not been properly inactivated and contained live, virulent poliovirus. It is highly unlikely that such an accident will be repeated.

ORAL POLIOVIRUS VACCINE

Oral polio vaccine (OPV), also referred to as poliovirus, live, oral, trivalent (TOPV), or Sabin vaccine) was first licensed for use in the United States in 1963. The primary vaccination series produces antibodies to all three serotypes in more than 95% of recipients; these antibodies remain for several years. As with IPV, recall boosters are recommended for maintaining adequate antibody levels.

The major advantages of OPV include ease of administration and the fact that the vaccine virus shed in the intestinal tract may result in secondary immunization of some nonimmune contacts of vaccinees. Also, it is theorized that during outbreaks the transient virus colonization and the induction of mucosal immunity may interfere with acquisition and spread of wild poliovirus. The importance of intestinal immunity induced by OPV is uncertain. The duration of significant local protection varies and its importance to the person or to public health control of wild poliovirus is a continuing subject for debate.

Like wild poliovirus, vaccine may be shed from the oropharynx for one to three weeks, and in the feces for six weeks or longer.

RATIONALE FOR ACTIVE IMMUNIZATION

Since there is little or no cross-immunity between the three poliovirus serotypes, trivalent OPV or IPV is used in all routine immunization programs. Major policy-making groups (committees of the American Academy of Pediatrics, the United States Public Health Service, and the National Academy of Sciences) currently recommend OPV for primary immunization of infants and children, with IPV reserved for adult immunization and other special circumstances. These committees cite the advantages noted for OPV, as well as the experience with it over the past two decades in the nearly total eradication of wild poliovirus infection.

However, in some countries, particularly the Scandinavian countries, a remarkable record of poliomyelitis control has been achieved with the exclusive use of IPV. The major arguments have centered around the issues of *herd immunity* (ability to reach a significantly large proportion of the population for primary immunization versus reliance on secondary spread of OPV to nonvaccinated persons and induction of local intestinal immunity to limit spread of wild virus strains), vaccine acceptance, and availability of adequate supplies of IPV. This last issue may be the major limiting factor in the immediate future.

Proponents of IPV point out the successes of programs that have relied exclusively on that vaccine, as well as its relative safety as compared with OPV.

Clearly, either vaccine, when given at the recommended doses and intervals, is effective in inducing protective immunity (Fig. 12-3). Vaccine recipients or their parents should be informed of the two types of vaccines available and the reasons why each is recommended. In addition, the risks and benefits of these vaccines to the individual and to the community should be stated so that a fully informed choice can be made before vaccination (see Chap. 3).

IMMUNITY

Protective immunity correlates with the presence of circulating neutralizing antibodies to all three poliovirus serotypes. Both OPV and IPV can readily induce antibody production which can be detected as early as three days after immunization. Peak antibody titers usually develop within two to four weeks and persist at lower levels for periods ranging to eight years or longer. Five years after a primary immunization series, antibodies to type 1 can be detected in 92% to 98% of recipients, to type 2 in 98%, and to type 3 in 84% to 87%. Even when antibody titers fall to undetectable levels, protection may exist, because reimmunization usually provokes a vigorous, rapid, anamnestic antibody rise. However, to ensure continuing protection, periodic revaccination is recommended.

The role of cell-mediated immunity (CMI) induced by immunization is uncertain. The local intestinal immunity induced by OPV, which may consist of both specific secretory IgA antibody and localized CMI mech-

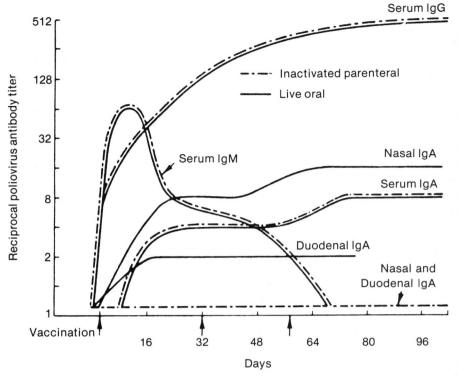

Fig. 12-3. Serum and secretory antibody response to orally administered live attenuated polio vaccine and to intramuscular innoculation of inactivated polio vaccine. (Ogra PL, Fishaut M, Gallagher MR: Viral vaccination via the mucosal routes. Rev Infect Dis 2:352–369, 1980; reprinted with permission of authors and publishers)

anisms, is known to develop but the duration and overall significance of this resistance is not known.

SCHEDULING OF POLIOVIRUS IMMUNIZATION

ROUTINE PRIMARY IMMUNIZATION FOR INFANTS, CHILDREN, AND ADOLESCENTS (UP TO 18th BIRTHDAY)

Oral Poliovirus Vaccine

The primary OPV series consists of *three* doses—the first two 6 to 8 weeks apart and the third by 8 to 12 months after the second. In infants, the series can be integrated with the diphtheria-tetanus-pertussis (DTP) vaccination, commencing at 6 to 12 weeks of age.

Inactivated Poliovirus Vaccine

The primary IPV series includes *four* doses—the first three 4 to 8 weeks apart and the fourth 6 to 12 months after the third. As with OPV, infant schedules can be integrated with the DTP vaccination.

IMMUNIZATION OF INFANTS AND CHILDREN WHO FAIL TO BE IMMUNIZED ACCORDING TO ROUTINE SCHEDULE

If a scheduled immunization is missed, the series for either OPV or IPV is resumed *without* a need to give additional doses beyond the number recommended (see Table 5-1.)

Since 1968, a higher-potency IPV has been in use; thus, four doses of IPV administered after 1968 are considered a primary series. If a partial series was given before then, the patient may need additional doses to ensure an adequate antibody response.

RECALL IMMUNIZATIONS

Oral Poliovirus Vaccine

At or just before school entry, any child who has received a three-dose primary OPV series should be given a fourth dose. Further boosters (actually, repeat doses of OPV are not true booster doses, but are intended to primarily immunize anyone who failed to respond to any of the three types following a previous immunization) beyond this are not now recommended except if the patient may later be at increased risk of exposure to wild poliovirus.

Inactivated Poliovirus Vaccine

At school entry, any child who received a four-dose primary IPV series should be given a fifth dose, to be repeated every five years until the child is 18-years old. Booster doses beyond this are not recommended unless there is increased risk of exposure.

IMMUNIZATION FOR ADULTS

In general, routine primary immunization of those beyond 18 years of age in the United States is neither indicated nor necessary. However, vaccination is recommended for those who may be at significant risk of exposure, such as health-care workers, certain laboratory employees, travelers to endemic or epidemic areas, or those who might be exposed to proven cases of poliomyelitis through family or community contact.

In these situations *IPV* is preferred because the risk of OPV-associated paralytic complications is slightly greater in adult patients than in infants or children. Oral polio vaccine should be used only if time does not permit adequate IPV immunization before the anticipated exposure.

An unvaccinated adult patient should be given three doses of IPV at 1 to 2 month intervals followed by a fourth dose 6 to 12 months later. Two doses of IPV are thought to afford reasonable initial protection, if time is a consideration, with completion of the series to continue as planned. If protection is needed more quickly because of epidemic exposure or plans to travel in 4 weeks or less, for example, a single dose of OPV is recommended.

Any adult patient who has previously received a partial IPV or OPV series may continue to receive the remaining doses of either vaccine regardless of the interval involved; anyone who has previously completed a primary series may be given booster doses of either IPV or OPV.

SPECIAL CIRCUMSTANCES

"Mixing and Matching"

In general, the same type of vaccine is used throughout an immunization series. However, if for reasons of availability or preference, one wishes to substitute IPV or OPV (or *vice versa*) in a primary series or booster regimen, there is no evidence to indicate that any impairment of immunologic responses or any adverse effects will occur.

Simultaneous Administration with Other Vaccines

Both OPV and IPV have been shown to be effective in inducing an antibody response when given *simultaneously* with certain other killed or live vaccines in various combinations. These include: (1) OPV or IPV with diphtheria-tetanus-pertussis vaccine, diphtheria-tetanus vaccine, or tetanus-diphtheria, adult type; and (2) Measles, mumps, rubella (combinations or singly), with the third or fourth dose of OPV (See Chap. 13 for further details.).

Breast Feeding and Oral Poliovirus Vaccine

Although poliovirus-neutralizing antibody can be detected in human colostrum, its inhibitory effect on OPV immunization appears to be significant only in the first postpartum week. After that, there is no reason to be concerned about the effectiveness of OPV in breast-fed infants, and timing of vaccine administration with respect to feeding schedules is not critical.

Unvaccinated Parents of Infants to be Given Oral Poliovirus Vaccine

While the risk of developing vaccine-associated paralysis in nonimmune parents of OPV recipients is remote, it is a concern to some health-care workers. One can elect to give the previously unimmunized adult two doses of IPV four weeks apart before initiating the OPV series in the infant; however, immunization of that infant should not be jeopardized or unduly delayed by such procedures. Some authorities recommend OPV for the infant without reference (or action) to the immune status of adults in the environment.

EPIDEMIC CONTROL

If there is a household case or community outbreak of presumed or proven poliomyelitis, OPV should be given to *all* potential contacts who have not been completely immunized or whose immunization status is unknown, except for persons who are immunodeficient. Theoretically, OPV is better than IPV in an epidemic, because it may interfere quickly with intestinal infection by wild poliovirus strains; however, proponents of IPV correctly point out that this has not been proved to be an advantage, and the appearance of protective circulating antibodies is similar for both vaccines.

PREMATURE INFANTS

Recently, the Academy of Pediatrics Committee on Infectious Diseases recommended using OPV in premature infants who are 2 months old and are being discharged from the hospital. They do not recommend using OPV when the infant must remain in the hospital after vaccination. Thus, for long hospitalization, DTP will be administered at the usual times and OPV initiated on the day of discharge. This recommendation is intended to avoid any spread of OPV viruses within the premature nursery or other pediatric inpatient unit.

SIDE-EFFECTS AND ADVERSE REACTIONS OF POLIOVIRUS VACCINES

INACTIVATED POLIOVIRUS VACCINE

No adverse effect has been reported for the currently available IPV preparations. Since they do contain trace amounts of streptomycin and neomycin, there is a remote possibility of hypersensitivity reactions in persons sensitive to these antibiotics.

ORAL POLIOVIRUS VACCINE

Vaccine-associated paralytic disease is a concern when OPV is used, and can occur in vaccine recipients or in their close contacts. The incidence is estimated at 1 in approximately 3.7 million doses distributed. In the United States, present estimates of vaccine-associated cases seen annually average approximately 4.3 per year. Of the 76 cases reported in the decade from 1969 to 1978, 18 were in otherwise healthy vaccine recipients, 47 in healthy close contacts, and 11 in persons with immune deficiency conditions. Aside from this last group, the risk of such a complication appears to increase with age; this is the primary reason why IPV is the preferred agent in unimmunized adult patients.

Transient suppression of tuberculin sensitivity, developing between 4 and 12 weeks after administration of monovalent type 1 OPV, has been reported. The sensitivity was regained in a few weeks and this has not been a problem in tuberculous patients on therapy.

SPECIFIC PRECAUTIONS

IMMUNODEFICIENCY

As with any live vaccine, OPV is strictly contraindicated for use in patients with proved or suspected immunodeficiency, *or* their household contacts. In addition, a family history should include inquiries about possible congenital immunodeficiency in close relatives, particularly before infant immunization is initiated. Besides the primary deficiency diseases, acquired states are also associated with an increased risk of vaccine-associated paralytic diseases including all malignancies, and other conditions in which therapy with corticosteroids, radiation, or antimetabolites have been used.

Such patients and their contacts can be safely vaccinated with IPV, and this is recommended.

PREGNANCY

Neither IPV nor OPV has been shown to have an adverse effect on the pregnant woman or her developing fetus; nevertheless, it is considered prudent to avoid any vaccinations in pregnancy, if at all possible. In urgent, epidemic-type exposures, however, OPV is recommended for previously unvaccinated women, whether pregnant or not.

REFERENCES

Bass JW, Halstead SB, Fischer GW et al: Oral polio vaccine. Effect of booster vaccination one to fourteen years after primary series. JAMA 239:2252–2255, 1978

Berkovich S, Starr S: Effects of live type 1 poliovirus vaccine and other viruses on the tuberculin skin test. New Engl J Med 274:67–72, 1966

Deforest A, Parker PP, Di Liberti JH et al: The effect of breast feeding on the antibody response of infants to trivalent oral poliovirus vaccine. J Pediatr 83:93–95, 1973

Fox JP: Eradication of poliomyelitis in the United States: A commentary on the Salk review. Rev Infect Dis 2:277–281, 1980

Immunization Practices Advisory Committee: Poliomyelitis prevention. Morb Mort Week Rep 28:510–520, 1979

John TJ, Devarajan LV, Luther L et al: Effect of breast feeding on seroresponse of infants to oral poliovirus vaccination. Pediatrics 57:47–53, 1976

Melnick JL: Advantages and disadvantages of killed and live poliomyelitis vaccines. Bull WHO 56:21–38, 1978

Nathanson N, Martin JR: The epidemiology of poliomyelitis: Enigmas surrounding its appearance, epidemicity, and disappearance. Am J Epidemiol 110:672–692, 1979

Nightingale EO: Recommendations for a national policy on poliomyelitis vaccination. New Engl J Med 297:249–253, 1977

Salk D: Eradication of poliomyelitis in the United States. III. Poliovaccines—practical considerations. Rev Infect Dis 2:258–273, 1980

Schonberger LB, Sullivan-Bolyai JZ, Bryan JA: Poliomyelitis in the United States. Adv Neurol 19:217–227, 1978

13

Combinations and Simultaneous Administration of Vaccines

Vincent A. Fulginiti

In the pure sense, the ideal immunization would be a highly defined antigen, given singly, once in a lifetime, and would confer 100% durable protection in all recipients. This ideal is seldom approached for most vaccines. Tempering achievement of this ideal is the practical need to minimize the number of both visits and injections and to ensure compliance and convenience. As a result, a rather constant goal among practical immunologists and physicians has been to combine vaccine antigens into compact doses that can be delivered at one time, or to simultaneously, but separately, administer vaccines. A few factors facilitate achievement of these procedures; others limit our approach to combining or simultaneously administering vaccines. The purpose of this chapter is to explore both generic and specific issues in these areas.

GENERAL CONSIDERATIONS

Combining some antigens may produce an unexpected benefit in that one antigen may act as an adjuvant for another in the combination. This is true for diphtheria-tetanus-pertussis (DTP) vaccine, as will be detailed later.

Convenience and economy of time make combined vaccinations advantageous. Also, the ability to offer protection against several diseases at once argues for such preparations and procedures. Finally, some persons and some populations have limited medical contact, and non-compliance is the rule. In these situations, the ability to administer multiple antigens on the few occasions that medical contact occurs is beneficial.

Limiting the combination of antigens in a single product is the potential for inactivation or reduction in potency of one or more components of the combined vaccine. Also, it is conceivable that side-effects and adverse reactions might be enhanced or additive if multiple products are administered. Finally, one does not wish to overwhelm the host's immunologic apparatus and to diminish the capacity to respond with an appropriate antibody or other immunologic response to individual components of the combined or simultaneously administered vaccines.

Thus, all combinations of individual vaccines must be scrupulously and thoroughly tested for effectiveness that is equivalent to single-antigen administration. In addition, the safety of the combined administration must be contrasted with that of the individual components. Sometimes, a compassionate physician believes that he is performing a great service for a patient by simultaneously administering multiple vaccines, sometimes in the same syringe. Often, he may do the patient a great disservice by such spontaneous combinations in that effectiveness may be reduced or adverse effects enhanced. *A solid general rule is that no combination of vaccines should be employed that has not been commercially prepared as a combination, licensed, and tested for both effectiveness and safety.*

In some instances of simultaneous but separate vaccine administration, there will be no extensive experience to guide the physician. Under these circumstances, the physician should follow the current recommendations summarized in the following sections. Some general guidelines will be discussed here that may prove useful in individual circumstances.

Inactivated vaccines can usually be administered simultaneously at separate sites. One must consider the side-effects anticipated from each and then judge the tolerance of the patient to simultaneously occurring local or systemic reactions. For example, if one gave DTP and cholera vaccine simultaneously, the resultant local and systemic reaction might prove unbearable. Thus such reactogenic vaccines should be given on separate occasions whenever possible. I have found that the need for simultaneous administration most commonly arises when foreign travel is anticipated. Whenever possible, regimens for administration of several vaccines in sequence should be carefully planned with the patient in order to permit enough time for appropriate, separate administration of the individual vaccines.

In similar fashion, an inactivated vaccine and a live virus vaccine can usually be administered simultaneously, but separately. The same precautions apply. Field-trial experience has indicated that some combinations, such as inactivated cholera vaccine and live yellow fever vaccine, should not be used.

Ordinarily, one would not wish to simultaneously administer single live virus vaccines. In general, one month's separation is recommended between doses of live virus vaccines. However, continuing observation suggests that neither effectiveness nor safety is reduced by the simultaneous administration of single live virus vaccines at separate sites. I believe that use of such simultaneous immunizations should be reserved only for situations of extreme need. If time and circumstance of disease exposure permit, separate administrations at least a month apart should be planned.

As new vaccines are introduced we must be alert for specific recommendations concerning their simultaneous use with other vaccines. Not all antigens can be expected to behave alike and some will not be usable for simultaneous administration.

If gamma globulin or other forms of passive antibody are administered, then live virus vaccination should be delayed for three months. For some diseases, simultaneous administration of serum or immune globulin and inactivated vaccines is recommended. In these circumstances, the specific dosage and frequency of vaccine administration may be altered because antibody has been simultaneously administered. Attention to these alterations is mandatory if the immunizing procedure is to achieve the desired effect. In the separate disease sections, whenever such simultaneous administration of antibody and antigen is contemplated, specific recommendations are made concerning alteration in vaccine usage.

SPECIFIC COMBINATIONS AND SIMULTANEOUS ADMINISTRATION OF VACCINES

DIPHTHERIA-TETANUS-PERTUSSIS VACCINE AND DIPHTHERIA-TETANUS VACCINE (PEDIATRIC AND ADULT)

Originally tested and administered as single antigens, the combinations of diphtheria and tetanus toxoids and pertussis vaccine have withstood the test of time. Each antigen is at least as antigenic in the combinations as if given alone, and there is no cumulative toxicity or excess adverse effect. There is some evidence for enhancement of antibody response to diphtheria and tetanus toxoids because of the presence of pertussis bacilli, and possibly endotoxin, in DTP.

It should be understood that DTP is more reactogenic than either diphtheria-tetanus, pediatric type (DT) or tetanus-diphtheria, adult type (Td) owing to the predictable rates of reaction to pertussis vaccine (see Chap. 6, 7, and 8). However, there is no greater reaction rate to pertussis in DTP than if it were administered alone in the same form.

POLIOVIRUSES

Administration of all three types of polioviruses, either oral (OPV) or inactivated (IPV), does not diminish potency of any single type of poliovirus or enhance side-effects. In early trials of OPV, inclusion of too large a dose of type 2 live, attenuated poliovirus tended to overshadow responses to types 1 and 3. This effect was presumably secondary to type 2 poliovirus's capacity to infect a large number of mucosal cells preferentially. Adjustment of the amount of type 2 virus in relation to types 1 and 3 corrected this defect of the original combination. Each 0.5-ml dose of currently available OPV contains 800,000 $TCID_{50}$ for type 1, 500,000 for type 3, and only 100,000 for type 2.

DIPHTHERIA-TETANUS-PERTUSSIS VACCINE COMBINED WITH INACTIVATED POLIOVIRUS VACCINE

No longer available commercially in the United States, a combination of diphtheria-tetanus-pertussis and inactivated poliovirus (DTPP) was used for a short period in the 1960s. In some countries such as Canada, it is still available. In one batch of vaccine prepared in this fashion, the effectiveness of the pertussis component was diminished by the presence of IPV vaccine. This effect was believed to be due to the preservative used in the preparation of IPV and was corrected in subsequent preparations.

In the future, DTPP may become available again. If so, the specific combination will need to be checked for both effectiveness (of all components) and safety prior to licensing.

MEASLES, MUMPS, AND RUBELLA VIRUS VACCINES

These live, attenuated viruses are available in several combinations: measles-mumps-rubella (MMR), measles-rubella (MR) and mumps-rubella (MuR). Each of these combinations is produced under strict control to ensure that no inactivation occurs in preparation, in storage, or upon reconstitution. Field studies have demonstrated approximately equal effectiveness of each component of the vaccine as compared with single administration of each antigen. Further, no interference in immunologic responses among component viruses has been demonstrated. Finally, no increase in side-effects or adverse reactions has been encountered.

If each single vaccine is administered individually but separately and at a different site, there is no evidence of diminished effect or enhanced reactivity. However, spontaneously combining single vaccine preparations into the same syringe or administering three single vaccines at the same site is strongly discouraged. Such procedures may inactivate these fragile agents or otherwise interfere with their intended effectiveness.

SIMULTANEOUS ADMINISTRATION OF DIPHTHERIA-TETANUS-PERTUSSIS VACCINE, MEASLES-MUMPS-RUBELLA VACCINE, AND ORAL POLIOVIRUS VACCINE IN VARIOUS COMBINATIONS

Simultaneous administration of DTP by intramuscular injection and OPV by oral administration is recommended; the recipient responds to all six antigens without any adverse consequences.

Simultaneous administration of OPV by mouth and MMR by subcutaneous injection results in adequate antibody response to all six antigens without enhancement of side-effects.

The simultaneous administration of DTP, OPV, and MMR by appropriate routes has not been as extensively evaluated as other combinations of these vaccines. What little data exist suggest no diminution in potency for any of the nine antigens and no increase in side-effects over that expected for each component alone. I'm reluctant to accept a recommendation that DTP-OPV-MMR be given routinely; this combination should be reserved for use in those situations in which the recipient is unlikely to return frequently, *or* in populations where noncompliance is expected, *or* for nonimmune persons who have little time available for receipt of vaccine prior to expected exposure. The last instance usually applies to travelers to areas endemic for these childhood diseases.

INFLUENZA VACCINE AND PNEUMOCOCCAL POLYSACCHARIDE VACCINE

Efficient antibody stimulation to all components of these two vaccines given simultaneously (16 to 17 antigens) has been demonstrated in a few studies. These studies were accomplished only with whole, inactivated influenza virus vaccine and have not been demonstrated for split-product (subvirion) influenza vaccine. Analysis of this combination continues, and results of more recent studies have suggested that interference may in fact occur. As a result, I am unable to make a firm recommendation at this time for the combination of these two vaccines. Although use of this combination might find favor among populations in which respiratory disease represents a significant risk to health or life, it would appear prudent to administer the components separately until adequate data indicate that the simultaneous administration is without risk of diminished immunologic stimulation.

INACTIVATED CHOLERA VACCINE AND LIVE YELLOW FEVER VIRUS VACCINE

Simultaneous or near simultaneous (within three weeks) administration of these two vaccines can inhibit the response to both. Because these vaccines are often needed for a person traveling to an area where both diseases are endemic, the demonstrated antagonism strongly recommends against simultaneous administration.

OTHER COMBINATIONS OR SIMULTANEOUSLY ADMINISTERED VACCINES

Some unusual combinations of a variety of vaccines have been studied under specific conditions. For example, some years ago the combination of smallpox vaccine (vaccinia virus) and live measles virus (LMV) vaccine was found to be effective and safe when delivered simultaneously by jet injection into the skin and subcutaneous tissues. The need for this combination disappeared along with smallpox, and the indications for smallpox vaccination. Thus, although of historic interest and of biologic importance, this combination is not used today.

In Third World countries, it would be advantageous to consider combining LMV vaccine with meningococcal vaccines. One study involving 110 children between 8 months and 4 years of age demonstrated that the combination of LMV vaccine with meningococcal A vaccine, or with the combined A + C vaccine, did not interfere with the development of meningococcal antibodies. However, the reverse was not true. Meningococcal A and meningococcal A + C vaccine appeared to depress measles vaccine effectiveness. Only 80% of the children tested showed seroconversion to measles when measles vaccine was combined with meningococcus A, and only 69% when it was combined with meningococcal A + C vaccine.

There have been preliminary studies of the simultaneous administration by a single injection of a spontaneous mixture of measles, tetanus, and meningococcal vaccines. The results are somewhat clouded, and the effectiveness of this combination is uncertain. The data are insufficient to recommend use of this procedure.

In the past, a large number of combinations of vaccines have been used in limited field trials to assess the effectiveness of simultaneous administration. It is beyond the scope of this chapter to detail each and every such effort. It is sufficient to note that none of these multiple combinations has achieved practical use anywhere in the world, except for those noted in the separate sections above. Further research might demonstrate that combinations of multiple vaccines not currently employed might be useful in certain situations, particularly in areas of both disease endemnicity and limited access to health care.

One final consideration is the possibility of inhibition of the vaccines that are administered sequentially but not simultaneously. As has been noted for cholera and yellow fever vaccines, near simultaneous administration may result in inhibition of adequate immunologic responses to either antigen. It has also been noted that LMV vaccine can inhibit smallpox virus replication if the LMV vaccine is given within a few days or weeks prior to smallpox vaccination. For these reasons, intervals between immunizations have been determined for many of the common vaccines. These intervals are indicated in this text in both the general sections and in specific disease and vaccine descriptions. The practitioner is urged to conform to these intervals in order to avoid failure in immunoprophylaxis.

REFERENCES

Barkin RM, Pichichero ME: Diphtheria-pertussis-tetanus vaccine: Reactogenicity of commercial products. Pediatrics 63:256–260, 1979

Brown GC, Volk VK, Gottshall RY et al: Responses of infants to DTP-P vaccine used in nine injection schedules. Publ Health Rep 79:585–601, 1964

Center for Disease Control. General recommendations on immunization. Morb Mort Week Rep 29:76, 81–83, 1980

Cluff LE, Allen JA: Principles of active immunization for prevention of infection. J Chron Dis 15:575–587, 1962

Edsall G: Application of immunological principles to immunization practices. Med Clin North Am 49:1729–1756, 1965

Edsall G, McComb JA, Wetterlow LH et al: Significance of the loss of potency in the pertussis component of certain lots of "quadruple antigen". New Engl J Med 267:687–689, 1962

Felsenfeld O, Wolf RH, Gyr LS et al: Simultaneous vaccination against cholera and yellow fever. Lancet 1:457–458, 1973

Hilleman MR: Experiences with combined viral vaccines. Symp Series Immunobiol Stand 7:7–20, 1967

Marks MI, Brazeau M, Shapera RM: Immunization today—a review. Can Med Assoc J 108:1413–1418, 1973

McBean AM, Gateff G, Manelark CR et al: Simultaneous administration of live attenuated measles vaccine with DTP vaccine. Pediatrics 62:288–291, 1978

Meyer HM Jr, Hostetler DD Jr, Bernheim BC et al: Response of Volta children to jet inoculation of combined live measles, smallpox and yellow fever vaccines. Bull WHO 30:783–789, 1964

Middaugh JP: Side effects of diphtheria-tetanus toxoid in adults. Am J Pub Health 69:246–249, 1979

Petersen JC, Christie A: Immunization in the young infant: Response to combined vaccines. Am J Dis Child 81:483–486, 1951

Phillips CF: Children out of step with immunization. Pediatrics 55:877 1975

Ruuskanen O, Viljanen MK, Salmi TT et al: DTP and DTP-inactivated polio vaccines. Acta Paediatr Scand 69:177–182, 1980

Weibel RE, Stokes J Jr, Buynak EB et al: Clinical-laboratory experience with combined dried live measles smallpox vaccine. Pediatrics 37:913–920, 1966

14
Smallpox

Vincent A. Fulginiti

This description of smallpox and smallpox vaccine is included despite the fact that there are no indications for its use at present. In spite of this recommendation, smallpox vaccine continues to be used by some practitioners, and is being used routinely in the military. For these reasons and for historical interest, this chapter is included in this text. This chapter is specially dedicated to C. Henry Kempe, M.D., who labored long and hard for the eradication of both smallpox and vaccination.

Smallpox no longer occurs anywhere in the world. Since October 1977, there has been no known case of natural smallpox, despite stringent and rigorous efforts to identify infection. The global eradication of smallpox was the result of an intensive campaign of case-finding and application of immunization with smallpox vaccine in the remaining endemic foci in the world prior to 1977.

The residual smallpox virus is limited to six research laboratories under strict supervision. There has been one instance of transmission of the virus in such a laboratory, underscoring the need for vigilance in handling the virus. In 1981, there should be no need to immunize anyone in the world against smallpox.

DISEASE

Smallpox is caused by a large DNA virus with widespread systemic manifestations. Smallpox occurs only in humans with no known animal reservoir. It is transmitted from human to human, probably by the respiratory route.

Clinical smallpox occurs following an asymptomatic incubation period lasting from 8 to 16 days. The disease has several phases. The prodromal phase is characterized by the sudden onset of high fever, severe headache, back pain, and vomiting. Following the prodromal phase, there may be a period of well being, or the disease may progress inexorably into the next stage. The second clinical phase is characterized by the appearance of the typical eruption. Macules appear first, developing within hours into firm nodular papules that vesiculate in 5 to 7 days. Early in the second week of illness, the vesicles become pustules as large as 1 cm in diameter. The rash begins distally on the extremities and progresses toward the trunk with sparing of the axilla. In discrete forms of the disease, the concentration of lesions on the trunk is smaller than that on the extremities. In some cases, enanthems may develop with painful punched-out ulcers appearing on the buccal mucosa, the palate, and the pharynx.

Smallpox has many variations ranging from an acute, fulminant hemorrhagic illness that may be lethal, to a very mild illness in which only a few pox lesions appear. For a more complete description of these manifestations of the disease, the reader is referred to Dixon and Fulginiti's descriptions in the references at the end of this chapter.

The mortality rate from smallpox varies from less than 1% in the mild forms of the disease to virtually 100% in the fulminant, hemorrhagic form. The infection involves many organs and systems, and considerable permanent disability and disfigurement may result from this acute infection.

IMMUNIZING ANTIGEN

As noted in Chapter 1, the modern immunizing antigen used to prevent smallpox was originally derived from cowpox. The origins of vaccinia virus are confused because numerous transfers and preparations have been made over the years. Some believe that the current virus was derived directly from cowpox and others believe that it is a laboratory variant that was attenuated by subsequent passage. Vaccinia virus is derived from dermal infection of calves with harvest of the resulting confluent lesions. The vaccine is partially clarified and prepared in individual or multiple-dose forms. There have been some attempts to adapt the vaccine to eggs and chick embryo tissue culture, and in the past preparations from both sources were available. These preparations are now only of historic interest, because the vaccine is no longer routinely recommended for anyone.

RATIONALE FOR ACTIVE IMMUNIZATION

Since the eradication of smallpox in 1977, there has been a gradual diminution in the indications for smallpox immunization. Soon after the last case was recorded, health workers, others who might have been exposed to smallpox virus in the laboratory, and members of the military were recommended as recipients of smallpox vaccine. In 1980, even these few recommendations were discontinued by the World Health Organization (WHO); however, the military continues to vaccinate active-duty personnel. *No one should receive smallpox vaccine except for those limited numbers of workers in the six laboratories in the world in which smallpox virus is still maintained.*

A few countries still require proof of smallpox immunization in order to gain entry. The WHO has indicated that a letter from a physician stating that a contraindication to vaccination exists should be honored by all countries. However, in practice, these recommendations are often not heeded and travelers may find that quarantine or immunization at a border site is demanded prior to entry. I hope that the few remaining bastions of conservatism concerning smallpox immunization will be overcome and that no traveler will experience any problems concerning smallpox immunization status.

The indications for smallpox immunization in the past were based upon the observation that vaccinia virus infection induced specific immunity in the recipient which prevented smallpox or modified its effects. Universal immunization was the rule in an effort to protect infants and to halt the spread of the disease.

In addition to individual immunization, selective primary immunization and reimmunization were carried out whenever smallpox was imported from an endemic part of the world to a nonendemic area. Known contacts were immunized in tier fashion; this practice of "ring" immunization of those who had been exposed to primary or secondary cases served to eliminate the massive immunization campaigns of the past. For example, in the late 1940s, with the importation of smallpox into New York City, millions of persons were immunized. In contrast, in the more recent importations to Europe, a much smaller circle of contacts was immunized, effectively halting the spread of smallpox. Should smallpox reappear for any reason, it is likely that immunization will take the ring form. It is extremely unlikely that smallpox will recur. A recent extensive analysis of this problem by Breman and Arita is recommended to readers who wish to pursue the matter further (see References).

IMMUNITY AGAINST SMALLPOX

Both variola and vaccinia viruses evoke complex sets of interactions in the infected host. Systemic antibodies, measurable in many different ways, can be regularly detected after infection. However, antibodies alone do not seem to be responsible for the limiting of virus replication and recovery from the initial episode. Cell-mediated immunity (CMI), mediated by the sensitized small lymphocyte (T cell), appears to be responsible for eradicating the disease. A multitude of animal and human studies have confirmed the central role of CMI. In fact, vaccinia virus still serves as a laboratory model for the study of CMI.

In addition, individuals with deficient CMI function experience severe progressive vaccinia virus infections, as will be detailed later. This indirect evidence also supports the view that CMI is most important in limiting and eradicating the virus.

In contrast, persons with B-cell deficiencies, unable to mount antibody responses to the vaccinia virus, have undergone normal vaccination without complications. This clinical observation also confirms the fact that antibodies do not have a significant role in recovery from acute infection. However, the presence of serum antibody appears to be correlated with a resistance to reinfection at some point in the future. The exact mechanism for this resistance to reinfection is not clear. It is also uncertain what role, if any, CMI plays in resisting reinfection with variola or vaccinia virus.

SCHEDULING OF SMALLPOX IMMUNIZATION

We will not detail former methods of immunization against smallpox here. For the interested reader, the references at the end of this chapter detail the mechanics of immunization and reimmunization.

SIDE-EFFECTS OF SMALLPOX VACCINATION

In the past, local side-effects of smallpox vaccination have included the production of local pustules and, on occasion, regional adenopathy. On rare occasions, the vaccination site became superinfected with bacteria, resulting in local staphylococcal or streptococcal impetiginous lesions. In some areas of the world where poultices were applied to the site of smallpox vaccination, tetanus was a complication. Such poultices were often contaminated with fecal material containing *Clostridium tetani* spores and the disease was transmitted through the open wound created by vaccination.

As many as 10% of those vaccinated experience erythema multiformlike eruptions that are noninfectious and are believed to be related to hypersensitivity to vaccinia virus or some other component of the vaccine. This generalized eruption is pruritic, lasting a few hours to several days.

ADVERSE SIDE-EFFECTS

In some cases, a generalized eruption develops after vaccinia virus is implanted in a local lesion (generalized vaccinia). These generalized, pox-like lesions are infectious and may be secondary to subtle immunologic unresponsiveness in the host. Selective absence of IgM has been suspected of predisposing to generalized vaccinia, although this finding has not been universal. This complication is benign and limited in duration; often only one or two successive crops of lesions are observed.

Progressive local lesions with viremic spread to many sites of the body may occur in persons with severely impaired T-cell function. Infants with severe combined immunodeficiency or with T-cell deficiencies, either congenital or acquired, experience progressive vaccinia (vaccinia necrosum). This potentially lethal disease has been well characterized (see References).

Vaccinia encephalitis occurs approximately once for each 50,000 primary vaccinations. Convulsions, lethargy, coma, paralysis, signs of cerebral edema and increased intracranial pressure, and focal neurologic findings are all observed in this complication.

On occasion, vaccinia virus is transferred from the site of original implantation to other parts of the body, resulting in secondary lesions (autoinoculation). These range from mild, limited disease to severe and extensive illness such as occurs in patients with eczema with transfer of the virus to abnormal skin, resulting in widespread eruption with up to 30% mortality.

In rare cases, the virus is transmitted transplacentally. Congenital vaccinia results in disseminated lesions; the infant is often stillborn or has extensive lesions at, or shortly after, birth.

REFERENCES

Breman JG, Arita I: The confirmation and maintenance of smallpox eradication. New Engl J Med 303:1263–1273, 1980

Center for Disease Control: Smallpox vaccine. Morb Mort Week Rep, 29:417–420, 1980

Dixon CW: Smallpox. London, Churchill, 1962

Fulginiti VA: Poxvirus diseases. In Kelley VC, Brennemann R (ed): Practice of Pediatrics. Hagerstown, Harper & Row, 1981

Fulginiti VA, Kempe CH, Hathaway WE et al: Progressive vaccinia in immunologic deficient individuals. In Bergsma D (ed): Immunologic Diseases in Man. New York, The National Foundation for March of Dimes, 1968

Goldstein JA, Neff JM, Lane JM et al: Smallpox vaccination reactions, prophylaxis and therapy of complications. Pediatrics 55:342–346, 1975

Karzon DT: Smallpox vaccination in the United States: The end of an era. J Pediatr 81:600–608, 1972

Kempe CH: Studies on smallpox and complications of smallpox vaccination. Pediatrics 26:172–189, 1960

Lane JM, Ruben ML, Neff JM et al: Complications of smallpox vaccination, 1968 J Infect Dis 122:303–309, 1970

Neff JM, Lane JM, Pert JH et al: Complications of smallpox vaccination. New Engl J Med 276:125–132, 1967

Wehrle PF: Smallpox eradication. A global appraisal. JAMA 240:1977–1979, 1978

World Health Organization. Weekly Epidemiologic Record 55:33–40, 121–128, 145–152, 153–160, 1980

15
Rabies

H. Robert Harrison

Rabies is an acute viral disease and is almost always transmitted to humans by the bite of an infected animal. After a variable incubation period, during which it multiplies locally, the virus gains entry into peripheral nerves, migrates cephalad, and produces a meningoencephalomyelitis that is almost invariably lethal.

There is no consistently effective treatment for clinical rabies. Prevention of disease following infection has depended upon pre- or postexposure prophylaxis with vaccination and passive antibody, and that, historically, has been unpleasant and dangerous in itself. Faced with a high case–fatality rate on the one hand, and an odious vaccine on the other, it is little wonder that physicians have found decisions about animal bite cases to be an unending agony.

Fortunately, major recent developments in rabies prophylaxis promise to render the clinician's decision making easier and to result in safer treatment.

DISEASE

The usual source of human infection is the saliva of rabid animals. Inoculation of rabies virus by a bite or salivary contamination of injured skin or intact mucous membranes may lead to clinical disease. Transmission from human to human through infected saliva, although theoretically possible, has not been documented. Other rare pathways of spread to humans have included airborne transmission from bat guano aerosols in caves, transmission from infected tissue or cells in laboratories, and transmission via corneal transplant. Rabies antigen has been recovered from human eye tissue. There have been a few cases in which a significant exposure could not be identified; since 1978, four such cases

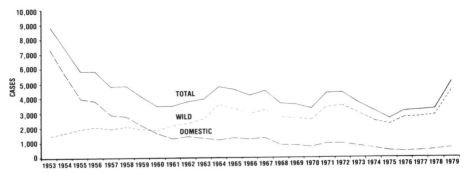

Fig. 15-1. Rabies: reported cases in wild and domestic animals by year, United States, 1953–1979. A total of 5119 laboratory-confirmed cases of animal rabies in the United States and 26 in Puerto Rico were reported in 1979. This was an increase from 1978 of more than 1800 cases, approximately a 67% gain from the average for the preceding 5 years. In fact, this is the largest number of cases reported since 1956. The District of Columbia, Hawaii, Idaho, Guam, and the Virgin Islands were the only areas reporting no rabies cases. Thirty-five states reported more cases of rabies in 1979 than in 1978, and 14 states and Puerto Rico reported less. Seven types of animals accounted for 98% of the reported cases. (Center for Disease Control. Morb Mort Week Rep, 28:54, 1980 [Annual Summary 1979])

of human rabies have occurred. The patient's inability to communicate exposure at the time of diagnosis is a possible explanation, although as yet undetermined routes may be responsible. The more recently identified transmission routes demand awareness from clinicians. Persons with progressive neurologic illness of unknown cause are not appropriate transplant donors. Rabies should always be considered in the differential diagnosis of meningoencephalitis of unknown cause, with features suggestive of this disease.

Animal bites are the most common route of rabies transmission. Depending on local epidemiology of rabies, the species of animal, and the site and severity of the bite, the mortality risk to the human will range from 0 to 100%; the average risk is estimated at 15%.

There are two reservoirs of virus: (1) sylvatic, occurring primarily among wild biting animals; and (2) urban, infecting dogs, cats, and other pets. Over the last 20 to 25 years, the incidence of rabies in the urban cycle has decreased dramatically, while that recorded in the sylvatic cycle has increased markedly. Bites of dogs, cats, and farm animals are rarely sources of rabies, while those of bats, skunks, foxes, coyotes, and bobcats are considered rabid exposures unless proven negative by brain examination. Rabid dogs still inhabit areas bordering

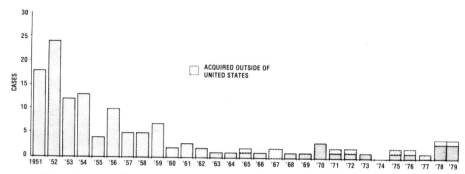

Fig. 15-2. Rabies: reported cases (registered deaths, 1951–1961) in humans by year, United States, 1951–1979 (Center for Disease Control. Morb Mort Week Rep, 28:54, 1980 [Annual Summary 1979])

Mexico, particularly El Paso/Juarez, and exposures in these regions are regarded as rabies-prone.

Rabies is not considered to be endemic in rodents in the United States; despite more than 24,000 rodent bites annually, no case of rabies has ever resulted. However, in recent years, a few rare rodents have been found which have been infected with rabies virus.

The incidence of rabies in humans in the United States has decreased from an average of 22 cases annually 30 years ago to one to five annually since 1960. The incidence in dogs has also dropped about 60-fold in that time. Although the likelihood of a significant dog or cat exposure is minimal, it is this type of exposure that still prompts 80% of antirabies treatment.

New Mexico has attempted to deal with the problem of unnecessary vaccination by establishing a comprehensive consultation-biologics system. Under this program, begun in September 1977, the New Mexico State Epidemiology Unit has provided: (1) treatment consultation to all state physicians 24 hours a day, 7 days a week; (2) coordination of rabies diagnosis and animal quarantine through the state laboratory and local animal control facilities; (3) free vaccine and antiserum to requesting physicians *regardless* of the epidemiology unit's treatment recommendations; (4) education of physicians about rabies treatment, epidemiology, and biologics; and (5) consultation on reactions and side-effects of biologics, and processing of titers to determine immune response.

During the first year of the program, there were 144 physician-initiated consultations and approximately 20% led to a decision to treat. This reduced approximately fivefold the number of postexposure prophylaxis courses given over previous years. If programs such as this were implemented throughout the United States, we could expect substantial physician education about rabies, and a reduction in the number and overall medical cost of postexposure treatments.

PATHOGENESIS AND IMMUNOLOGY

In most cases of peripheral bites, the virus remains at the site for up to 2 weeks and multiplies in muscle but it probably invades nervous tissue early. The virus is believed to spread to the central nervous system (CNS) along peripheral nerves; hematogenous infection is probably uncommon, if it occurs at all. Infection is almost certain if the virus makes direct contact with nerve tissue. In part, this phenomenon may explain the frequency, rapidity, and severity of infection following bites about the head and neck.

The prolonged incubation and symptom-free periods (10 days to 1 year) in rabies are not understood. The usual incubation period is 3 to 8 weeks. The ensuing encephalitis involves the brainstem and spinal cord to a greater degree than it does other sites in the CNS.

In animals, antibody is produced in response to infection that can be measured by neutralizing, complement-fixing, precipitating, hemagglutination inhibiting, and cytolytic tests. Neutralizing antibody is the basis of vaccine-induced immunity; a titer of more than 1 : 16 is believed to be highly correlated with protection.

Prevention of rabies depends upon either preexposure prophylaxis in identifiable high-risk persons or prompt and early postexposure prophylaxis during the asymptomatic period. Protection depends upon production of antibody against the virus prior to onset of disease. This is accomplished through a combination of active (vaccine) and passive (immune globulin) immunization. This regimen provides early passive immunity as a result of the immune globulin (IG), with active immunity developing later in response to the vaccine. Historically, equine hyperimmune rabies serum (RIS) was used for passive immunization but was attended by two problems. The first was that the serum sometimes interfered with the development of active vaccine-induced immunity. This led to the addition of two booster doses of vaccine (duck embryo at that time) after the end of the usual series. The second problem was that serum sickness was a frequent sequela.

In the 1960s, human rabies immune globulin (HRIG) was developed. It is prepared from pools of plasma donors who have received pre- or postexposure vaccination and have developed reasonably high antibody titers. Clinical studies in the early 1970s showed that optimal passive and active immunity was obtained with 20 IU/kg of HRIG and a course of duck embryo vaccine (DEV). This regimen resulted in geometric mean serum titers of more than 1 : 6 by day 1 and of more than 1 : 50 by day 25 of an immunization course and was associated with the lowest number of immunization failures.

The recently developed human diploid cell rabies vaccine (HDCV) has proven to be a much safer and more immunogenic vaccine than DEV and has supplanted the latter in this country. When given in a schedule of 0, 3, 7, 14, and 28 days the new vaccine has been shown to produce protective antibody levels at ten days, with or without concurrent administration of IG.

RABIES VACCINE

Successful postexposure active immunization was first performed by Pasteur in 1885. His vaccine was a live attenuated virus developed by serial intracerebral passage in rabbits; it was lethal for animals when inoculated intracerebrally but was immunogenic when used peripherally. Although an unparalleled achievement, the vaccine often produced severe adverse reactions or resulted in prophylactic failure with bite wounds of the face and head.

The next major development was the use of formalin-inactivated virus originally obtained from infected animal nerve tissue (Semple-type vaccine). This is still in use in many parts of the world although not in the United States. It is approximately 80 to 90% immunogenic and is associated in itself with significant morbidity. One patient per 3500 vaccinated experiences neuroparalytic disease, and one in 35,000 dies. The myelin is the causative agent in these immunologic disorders; the patient produces antimyelin antibody which is destructive to his own tissue.

In 1957, DEV was substituted for Semple-type vaccine in the United States, and was the only vaccine available in this country until recently. Virus propagated in embryonic duck tissue is inactivated by beta-propiolactone. The DEV was developed in order to circumvent the use of brain tissue vaccines and to decrease the incidence of neurologic disease in recipients. Between 1958 and 1975, neuroparalytic reactions were reported in 21 of 512,000 DEV recipients, or in one in 24,400. These reactions included transverse myelitis in five cases, cranial or peripheral neuropathy in seven, and encephalopathy in nine. Although DEV represents a significant advance over nerve tissue vaccines, it is not benign. Virtually every recipient experiences pain, erythema, and induration. Systemic symptoms develop in approximately 33% and anaphylaxis in 1% of those vaccinated. The 21-dose vaccine course is an unpleasant and inconvenient experience, especially for children.

The development and release of HDCV produced by adapting the

Pitman-Moore strain of virus to WI-38 or MRC-5 cell lines has been a major advance in rabies immunoprophylaxis. One such vaccine is produced by 1' Institut Merieux, Lyon, France, and is prepared from the MRC-5 adapted virus inactivated with betapropiolactone. Another (Wyeth) is produced with the WI-38 adapted virus and is inactivated with tri(n)butyl-phosphate-Tween 80 and merthiolate, resulting in a subunit vaccine. These two products, by virtue of their increased purity and human cell origin, have resulted in fewer adverse reactions, and no neuroparalytic disease in initial experience.

Trials have shown that these vaccines are similar in terms of potency and safety and are a substantial improvement when compared with DEV. No one exposed to a proven rabid animal and treated with HDCV, with or without IG, has developed rabies. This is particularly impressive because, in several cases, immunization was not begun until 3 to 8 days, and in one case, 14 days, following exposure.

In the most recent studies in this country, a five-dose schedule plus RIG has been successfully employed as judged by antibody response. Reactions to HDCV, although experienced by 44% of recipients, have been primarily local and relatively trivial. Mild systemic reactions (headache, nausea, diarrhea) have developed in less than 20%. Only one serious reaction in 5000 vaccinees has been documented. No neuroparalytic events have been reported.

From June to September 1980, 2500 patients in the United States received HDCV. A total of 25,200 doses were distributed. Some newly described side-effects included the following:

> Systemic allergic reactions (hives, anaphylactic shock, etc.) were experienced by four patients (1:625 treated). Some had repeated reactions with subsequent doses.
>
> Fever and severe headache unassociated with signs of CNS disease were experienced by four patients (1:625 treated). Symptoms resolved within 24 hours and occasionally recurred after subsequent doses.
>
> Chills, diarrhea, malaise, headache, and fever were also experienced by some recipients. Local reactions (erythema, induration, and pain) were observed in less than 25% of recipients of HDCV.
>
> No deaths or encephalopathy have been reported.

The relative lack of potency of nervous tissue vaccines and DEV resulted in the use of simultaneous passive immunization with RIS. Originally of equine origin, RIS was associated with risk of serum sickness in 46% of subjects over 15 years of age and in 16% of all subjects. Equine RIS has been replaced in this country with HRIG, a potent and low-risk preparation prepared by cold ethanol fractionation from plasma of hyperimmunized human donors. Despite the demonstrated immunogenicity of the HDCV, passive immunization with HRIG is still performed.

SCHEDULING OF IMMUNIZATION

The Wyeth HDCV is not commercially available at present. However, under the terms of the patent held by the Wistar Institute, Wyeth has rights for commercial distribution of HDCV in North America. The Merieux vaccine, which became available in June 1980, originally was distributed only through federal, state, or local government agencies. Long-range plans include full availability from commercial sources. The vaccine is expensive and unaffordable in many parts of the world; hence we include recommendations for DEV and RIS as well as for HDRV and HRIG.

PRE-EXPOSURE PROPHYLAXIS

The low frequency of severe reactions to DEV and even lower frequency for HDCV makes pre-exposure prophylaxis practical for high-risk groups. These include veterinarians, animal handlers, laboratory workers exposed to rabies virus, and people living in or visiting countries in which rabies remains a constant peril and for whom rabies exposure by virtue of activity or residence is likely. Persons whose work or hobby puts them at high risk of contact with rabid animals such as foxes, skunks, bats, and coyotes should also consider pre-exposure immunization.

Prophylaxis in high-risk cases may provide protection against inapparent exposure to rabies. It also simplifies postexposure therapy by eliminating the need for HRIG and by decreasing the number of vaccine doses needed. This is especially important in countries or in situations where postexposure therapy may be delayed or where the vaccines available have a higher risk of sequelae.

Vaccines. If available, HDCV should be used. Three 1 ml intramuscular injections are given, one on each of days 0, 7, and 21 or 28. This regimen has been found to induce antibody in 98.4 to 100% of vaccinees, depending upon the serologic technique employed. It is suggested that serologic testing for rabies antibody titer be done 2 to 3 weeks after the last dose. If the response is inadequate (*i.e.,* less than 1 : 16) a booster dose should be administered and a repeat serum titer should be performed.

Alternatively, three 1 ml subcutaneous injections of DEV can be employed, the first two given 1 month apart and the third dose given 6 to 7 months after the second. If a more rapid schedule is desired, three 1 ml injections can be given at weekly intervals, with a fourth dose 3 months later. If serum antibody is less than 1 : 16, two booster doses 1 week apart can be given and repeat serum collected 2 to 3 weeks later.

Persons with a continuing risk of exposure should either have a 1 ml booster dose every 2 years or, alternatively, have a serum antibody level determined every 2 years with a booster dose if necessary.

A pre-immunized person with demonstrated antibody who is exposed to rabies should receive two doses of HDCV at 3-day intervals, or five daily doses of DEV plus a booster dose on day 25. Passive immunization is not necessary. If the antibody titer is not known, a serum sample should be immediately examined for antirabies titer and full postexposure treatment begun until the immune status is determined. Serum titers can be obtained through state health departments and the Center for Disease Control (CDC).

POSTEXPOSURE PROPHYLAXIS

Animal bites come to medical attention at an annual rate of one per 200 persons. This results in rabies vaccination for 30,000 persons per year. Approximately 80% of these series are unnecessary. Although HDCV seems to be a much more benign vaccine than DEV, indiscriminate use of this vaccine should not become a substitute for good clinical evaluation according to established guidelines. Recent experience with swine influenza vaccine, which appeared even more benign than HDCV, should caution about indiscriminate use of any new product. New Mexico health authorities have shown that the number of vaccine courses may be reduced fivefold without danger to patients by careful assessment of risk and appropriate use of diagnostic techniques as described in the foregoing. Finally, HDCV is quite expensive as compared with previous vaccines.

Several factors must be considered in combination in risk assessment: (1) the species of animal; (2) the circumstances of the incident; (3) the type of exposure; (4) the severity of exposure; (5) the location of the animal; (6) the rabies epidemiology in the region; and (7) the vaccination status of the animal.

Animals in the United States can be regarded as both high- and low-risk for transmission of rabies. In general, domestic animals such as dogs, cats and farm animals are of low risk. Wild animals, especially bats, skunks, foxes, coyotes, bobcats, racoons, and other carnivores should be regarded as high-risk in all circumstances. Rodents and rabbits are of very low risk, and for practical purposes are usually considered of no risk.

Any unprovoked attack by a domestic animal is more likely to indicate that the animal is rabid, so obtaining a careful history of the circumstances surrounding the biting incident is important. In general, bites that occur during feeding or handling of a healthy looking animal are considered as provoked. In cases involving children, it is often difficult to obtain an accurate history especially if an adult was not present when the bite occurred. *If in doubt about the circumstances, consider the attack unprovoked.* Any attack by a wild animal is a rabid exposure until proved otherwise.

The type of exposure is generally divided into bite and nonbite. A bite is any penetration of the skin by teeth. Nonbites consist of scratches, abrasions, open wounds, or mucous membranes contaminated by saliva from a rabid animal. Casual contact without a bite or nonbite exposure does not constitute an exposure. Human-to-human transmission has not been documented.

Animal bites are generally distributed in the following percentages: head, 5%; trunk, 5%; arm, 40%; and leg, 50%. Bites around the face, neck, and head are more likely to result in rabies. Deaths from facial bites occur 10 times and 28 times more frequently than do deaths from upper and lower limb bites, respectively. In general, more extensive lesions or multiple bites, especially with many puncture wounds, are regarded as more likely to result in disease.

An escaped animal is of more concern because quarantine or sacrifice is then not an option. The decision to use rabies prophylaxis then depends upon evaluation of other factors to determine the likelihood of a rabid exposure.

Regional epidemiologic data are available through state and local health departments. The recent occurrence of rabies (by animal examination) in the species involved in the incident is usually known. This is especially important if the animal has escaped, because it may dictate whether the exposure is high- or low-risk. Of particular relevance is the occurrence of rabies in stray dogs and cats involved in exposure within a given region or community, because this is the most common circumstance in which care is sought.

The vaccination status of the offending animal is of crucial importance. A mature animal, appropriately immunized with one or more doses of potent animal vaccines, is unlikely to develop rabies or to carry the virus in its saliva.

Examples of this combination approach are considered below to illustrate the above considerations in practical decision making.

Case 1. A 13-year-old girl is bitten on the left leg while riding a bicycle down a city street. The dog cannot be found, but was observed to have a collar with tags around its neck. There has been no rabies found in domestic dogs in that city for 10 years. On examination, there are two puncture wounds and several abrasions on the lateral calf.

In this case, local care and ascertainment of tetanus immune status are indicated, but not immunoprophylaxis for rabies. The animal is domestic, the attack provoked (dogs do not like bicycles). The animal has probably been licensed and vaccinated. Even if not, there is no dog rabies in the region. The exposure, although a bite, is at a relatively low-risk site.

Case 2. A 7-year-old boy is brought in with several bites on the right hand that he got the previous evening while cleaning his pet skunk's cage. The skunk has been in good health and was purchased from a local pet shop. Examination reveals several bite wounds on the fingers and dorsum of the hand.

This incident is considered a rabid exposure, as skunks are wild animals and rabies has occurred in "domesticated" animals sold by pet shops. Under these circumstances, the animal should be killed under appropriate conditions and the head examined for rabies antigen. Quarantine is inappropriate. Local state health officials, as well as veterinarians, will assist in coordinating the appropriate shipment and examination procedures. If the animal is rabid, postexposure prophylaxis ensues, and the pet shop is thoroughly investigated by public health officials. If the skunk is negative, no immunization is necessary.

Case 3. A 13-year-old girl is walking down the street in a city 75 miles from the Mexican border. An unknown dog on the other side of the street runs across, jumps up, and bites her on the arm, runs away and cannot be located. There has been no domestic animal rabies in this city or county for the previous four years, although there have been cases in close proximity to the border.

This case conveys the dilemma involved in many postexposure prophylaxis decisions. The exposure is unprovoked, the animal has escaped. The dog is probably domestic, but immunization status is unclear. There is, however, no known rabies in domestic animals in the city. If the physician were to rely on local epidemiology, this would be a nonrabid exposure and no immunization would be given. On the other hand, no physician wants to preside over the first case of dog rabies in that city in four years! Either decision, to treat or not to treat, must be considered correct. In either case, however, all possible efforts must be made in concert with local authorities to locate and observe the animal.

Postexposure prophylaxis consists of a triad of wound management, animal management, and induction of immunity.

Wound Management. Immediate and thorough washing of all bite and nonbite wounds is both important and very effective. Simple soap and water is preferred; benzalkonium chloride and nitric acid are neither indicated nor necessary. Tetanus prophylaxis and antibacterial therapy should be employed as indicated (see Chapter 8 on tetanus).

TABLE 15-1.   Rabies postexposure prophylaxis guide, March 1980

The following recommendations are only a guide. In applying them, take into account the animal species involved, the circumstances of the bite or other exposure, the vaccination status of the animal, and presence of rabies in the region. **Local or state public health officials should be consulted if questions arise about the need for rabies prophylaxis.**

	Animal Species	Condition of Animal at Time of Attack	Treatment of Exposed Person*
Domestic	Dog and cat	Healthy and available for 10 days of observation	None, unless animal develops rabies†
		Rabid or suspected rabid	RIG‡ and HDCV§
		Unknown (escaped)	Consult public health officials. If treatment is indicated, give RIG‡ and HDCV§
Wild	Skunk, bat, fox, coyote, raccoon, bobcat, and other carnivores	Regard as rabid unless proven negative by laboratory tests ¶	RIG‡ and HDCV§
Other	Livestock, rodents, and lagomorphs (rabbits and hares)	Consider individually. Local and state public health officials should be consulted on questions about the need for rabies prophylaxis. Bites of squirrels, hamsters, guinea pigs, gerbils, chipmunks, rats, mice, other rodents, rabbits, and hares almost never call for antirabies prophylaxis.	

* All bites and wounds should immediately be thoroughly cleansed with soap and water. If antirabies treatment is indicated, both rabies immune globulin (RIG) and human diploid cell rabies vaccine (HDCV) should be given as soon as possible, regardless of the interval from exposure.

† During the usual holding period of 10 days, begin treatment with RIG and vaccine (preferably with HDCV) at first sign of rabies in a dog or cat that has bitten someone. The symptomatic animal should be killed immediately and tested.

‡ If RIG is not available, use antirabies serum, equine (ARS). Do not use more than the recommended dosage.

§ If HDCV is not available, use duck embryo vaccine (DEV). Local reactions to vaccines are common and do not contraindicate continuing treatment. Discontinue vaccine if fluorescent-antibody (FA) tests of the animal are negative.

¶ The animal should be killed and tested as soon as possible. Holding for observation is not recommended.

Animal Management. As shown in Table 15-1, a healthy domestic dog or cat involved in a biting incident should be confined and observed for 10 days and evaluated by a veterinarian at the first sign of illness. If the animal falls ill or if signs suggestive of rabies develop, the animal should be killed and the head removed and shipped, under refrigeration, to a qualified laboratory for examination with prior communication to establish proper handling and shipping procedures. These laboratories are designated by state or local health departments. Any stray, unwanted, or initially ill animal should be killed immediately without quarantine and the brain examined.

Signs of rabies in wild animals are not reliable. Any wild animal biting or scratching a human should be killed and the brain examined. If the brain does not contain rabies antigen by fluorescent-antibody determination, the person need not be treated.

Care must be exercised in killing the animal in order to prevent biting or salivary contact by the handlers and to ensure that the brain is not injured (*e.g.*, don't shoot the animal in the head). Help from a professional such as a veterinarian or equivalent should be sought whenever feasible.

IMMUNIZATION

A useful summary is provided in Table 15-1. Postexposure treatment includes vaccine plus HRIG except in cases involving persons with documented adequate antirabies titers. The sooner treatment is begun, the more likely it is to be successful. If in doubt, initiate therapy with both HDCV and HRIG.

The HDCV is the vaccine of choice. In the United States, a five dose vaccine regimen is recommended (days 0, 3, 7, 14, and 28). Day 0 refers to the day of initiation of vaccination. (The WHO currently recommends a sixth dose at 90 days). A serum specimen for antibody titer should be collected on day 28. One dose of HRIG is given with the first dose of HDCV.

If HDCV cannot be obtained, DEV is used. One dose of HRIG and 23 doses of DEV are given. The DEV regimen can consist of 21 daily doses or of 14 doses in the first seven days (two injections at separate sites simultaneously) followed by seven daily single doses. The 22nd and 23rd doses are each given at 10-day intervals after the day of the 21st dose. Since DEV is a subcutaneous vaccine and local reactions are very common, rotation of sites (abdomen, back, thighs) is recommended. Antibody should be adequate and detectable by the time of the second booster dose. If not, administration of three doses of HDCV (days 0, 7, and 14) is imperative.

The HDCV can be used to complete immunization begun with DEV. After four to seven doses of DEV, use four doses of HDCV (days 0, 7, 14, and 28), and after eight or more doses, use three doses of HDCV (days 0, 7, and 14).

The HRIG is given only once at the start of therapy. If inadvertently omitted or unavailable, it can be given up to 8 days after the first vaccine dose. The quantity used is 20 IU/kg. Up to half of the total volume to be used should be infiltrated in the area surrounding the wound, and the remainder given intramuscularly.

If there is a high clinical suspicion of rabies after due consideration of a domestic stray animal bite, and the animal has escaped, it is wise to begin prophylaxis. In the event of capture, treatment can be terminated following uneventful quarantine or negative brain examination.

ACCIDENTAL EXPOSURE TO ANIMAL RABIES VACCINES

There are currently three modified live virus vaccines (MLV) used to immunize animals. Vaccine-associated rabies has occurred in animals given these precautions. The three MLV animal vaccines use HEP Flury, SAD, and Kissling virus strains. The HEP and SAD vaccines have been used for over 10 years without associated disease in exposed humans. Therefore, postexposure prophylaxis is not indicated. The Kissling vaccine has only been used since 1975, so experience is more limited. Although no human cases have been associated with its use, postexposure prophylaxis is recommended until further data are accumulated.

PRECAUTIONS AND CONTRAINDICATIONS

Steroids and immunosuppressive agents should not, if at all possible, be administered during postexposure treatment because they may interfere with active immunity. If they must be given, it is essential to test serum samples for development of adequate antirabies titer. Pregnancy is not a contraindication to either DEV or HDCV; both are inactivated vaccines.

REFERENCES

Alexander ER: Human diploid cell rabies vaccine: More protection for less risk? JAMA 244:816, 1980

Center for Disease Control: Human diploid cell rabies vaccine. Med Let 22:93–94, 1980

Center for Disease Control: Human rabies—Oklahoma. Morb Mort Week Rep 28:476–481, 1979

Center for Disease Control: Rabies prevention. Morb Mort Week Rep 29:265–279, 1980

Center for Disease Control: Two suspected cases of human rabies—Texas, Washington. Morb Mort Week Rep 28:292–298, 1979

Houff SA, Burton RC, Wilson RW et al: Human-to-human transmission of rabies virus by corneal transplant. New Engl J Med 300:603–604, 1979

Larghi OP, Nebel AE: Rabies virus inactivation by binary ethylenimine: New method for inactivated vaccine production. J Clin Microbiol 11:120– 122, 1980

Mann JM, Burkhart MJ, Rollag OJ: Anti-rabies treatments in New Mexico: Impact of a comprehensive consultation-biologics system. Am J Pub Health 70:128– 132, 1980

Plotkin SA, Wiktor T: Vaccination of children with human cell culture rabies vaccine. Pediatrics 63:219– 221, 1979

Spaeth R: Rabies. In Spittell JA (ed): Practice of Medicine, Vol 4, p 1– 27. Hagerstown, Harper & Row (in press)

16
Influenza

E. Russell Alexander

DISEASE

Influenza virus is the cause of annual epidemics with very high rates of illness and low mortality. Influenza is usually readily recognizable in communities by its ability to cause sharp epidemics of febrile respiratory disease in both children and adults—the epidemics usually lasting only 4 to 6 weeks. Although some influenza occurs each year, for any given location the incidence is extremely variable, and years of high incidence will be intermittent.

Infection may be asymptomatic or may cause mild to severe disease. Although the mortality rates are low, the almost universal occurrence of influenza over the span of a few years results in a large absolute number of deaths; influenza is one of the largest contributors to seasonal mortality. For example, in the period from 1968 to 1980, it is estimated that more than 150,000 excess deaths occurred due to influenza in the United States. Those succumbing are primarily infants and older patients (Fig. 16-1).

Apart from its contribution to mortality, the disease is important as an illness. No other epidemic disease can cause such sustained high absenteeism from school or from the workplace. The incidence is highest in school-age patients (5–19 years of age).

Characteristically, influenza causes a marked febrile illness (two-thirds of cases are symptomatic) with abrupt onset of chills, headache, anorexia, malaise, myalgias, and arthralgias. Upper respiratory symptoms follow, with lower respiratory tract involvement without pneumonia (such as tracheitis, bronchitis, bronchiolitis, and croup), primary influenza virus pneumonia, secondary bacterial pneumonia (most commonly pneumococcal), or concomitant viral and bacterial pneumonia. The nonpulmonary complications of influenza include en-

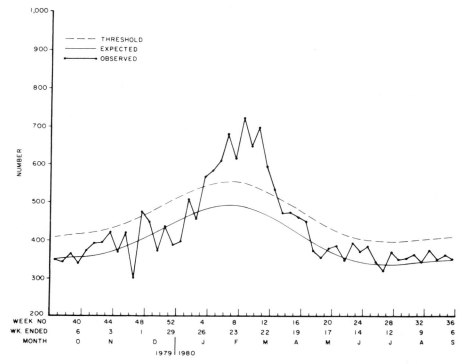

Fig. 16-1. Pneumonia-influenza: reported deaths in 117 selected cities by week, United States, September 1979– August 1980 (Center for Disease Control. Morb Mort Week Rep, 28:54, 1980 [Annual Summary 1979])

cephalitis, transverse myelitis, Guillain-Barre syndrome and Reye's syndrome (primarily following influenza B). Less commonly, pericarditis, myocarditis, pancreatitis, hemolytic-uremic syndrome, disseminated intravascular coagulation with renal failure, and myoglobinuria have been reported. An association of influenza and meningococcal mengitis has been recorded. It is uncertain whether influenza causes abortion, premature birth, or congenital malformations.

Influenza virus has three subtypes, A, B, and C, which differ both epidemiologically and clinically. Influenza A virus causes widespread pandemics and epidemics. High attack rates are observed in children and in adult patients with excess mortality consequent to antigenic variations in influenza virus antigenic structures.

Influenza A viruses are classified according to their hemagglutinin (H) and neuraminidase (N) antigens. To date, five subtypes of H and two of N have been recognized in the major antigenic shifts that have occurred (Fig. 16-2). With each major shift, worldwide pandemics have occurred.

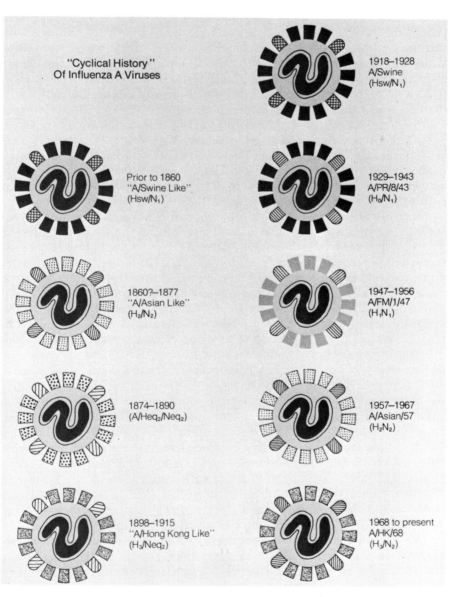

Fig. 16-2. "Cyclical history" of influenza A viruses (Carey L: U of Washington Med 4:12, 1977)

When a new variant develops, influenza spreads throughout the world in less than two seasons. The A/Swine strain ($H_{sw}N_1$) was introduced in 1918, and for the first two years of its existence, spread rapidly with extremely high mortality, especially among middle-aged patients. Minor antigenic changes (antigenic drift) occurred in subsequent years until another major shift occurred in 1929 with the introduction of H_0N_1 strains. H_1N_1 strains were introduced in 1947 and circulated until 1956. In 1957, the Asian strain heralded a new shift (H_2N_2). Since 1968, we have been undergoing a gradual shift of H_3N_2 strains following the Hong Kong variant pandemic. The most recent A strain, A/Bangkok/79, has drifted slightly from its predecessor A/Texas/77—both H_3N_2 strains.

The extent of occurrence of influenza, even in the intervening years between the pandemic years of a major shift, is reflected in the fact that within a few successive waves, the old antigenic strain is completely replaced by the new. For example, when the A/Port Chalmers (H_3N_2) variant (which caused disease in the United States through the autumn of 1975) was replaced by a new A/Victoria (H_3N_2) variant (which caused an epidemic in early January of that year), within one season no more A/Port Chalmers variants could be found in either the United States or elsewhere in the world including the most remote and isolated populations. Unlike swine, which harbor old strains (as they have the $H_{sw}N_1$ variants), we humans are more fickle and the old strain generally vanishes from the face of the earth. The speed of that replacement, nationally and internationally, indicates how quickly this agent spreads.

There have been two recent exceptions. In 1976, four isolates of a novel strain A/New Jersey/1976 ($H_{sw}N_1$) were recorded among recruits in training at Fort Dix, New Jersey. Serologic evidence showed a wider spread and it was estimated that approximately 400 recruits had become infected. Because a major antigenic shift was (and still is) anticipated, it was surmised that this had occurred. The theory that major antigenic shifts are not random events but follow a recycling pattern seemed to account for the emergence of the new swine strain. Serologic evidence suggests that strains similar to the 1968 Hong Kong strains (H_3N_2) existed in the period from 1898 to 1915 and that they were preceded by H_2N_2 strains. A pandemic of an $H_{sw}N_1$ strain was feared and in the United States, a massive effort resulted in the preparation and distribution of swine influenza vaccine, an effort now recognized as premature. In fact, even before that vaccine was distributed, it became clear that the A/New Jersey/1976 strain did not spread outside of the recruit camp. It represented a strain derived from swine which had the potential for epidemic spread but could not survive. There will undoubtedly be another major antigenic shift of influenza A virus in the next few years, but when and in what form remains unknown.

Another unusual event in recent years has been the resurgence of H_1N_1

strains. In November 1977, influenza was recognized in Moscow in outbreaks among persons under 22 years of age. It was identified as A/USSR/77 and was an H_1N_1 strain—a variant that had not caused influenza anywhere in the world for more than 20 years. This designation indicates that it was related to the strains that first appeared in Melbourne in 1946 and were the circulating strains until they were replaced by A/Asian/57 in 1957. In fact, the USSR strain (Russian flu) was most akin to the strains present in the early 1950s—a slight drift from the original. From 1977 to the present, the old rules have been broken and both H_3N_2 and H_1N_1 strains have caused epidemic influenza. The unique feature of the epidemiology of H_1N_1 influenza is that it has only occurred in those born before it was prevalent—and therefore only in the young, now defined as those less than 25 years of age. As the story became clearer, it was learned that the virus first appeared on the Sino-Russian border and had also been epidemic in China in 1977. The strain was also unique in that it grew readily in eggs, without adaptation, and therefore resembled a laboratory-adapted strain. Some have surmised that it escaped from a freezer rather than occurring through natural evolution. Nevertheless, it is still circulating in 1980. Whether it will continue to survive now that there are few susceptible persons is uncertain.

Influenza B virus undergoes less frequent antigenic variation, tends more often to cause localized outbreaks, produces fewer complications, and causes less mortality. It is more frequently associated with Reye's syndrome than is influenza A. Antigenic variation of B strains does occur and was noted most recently in the 1979–80 season when B/Singapore/79 became the predominant variant (a clear drift from the prior prototype B/Hong Kong/72).

Influenza C is mentioned only for the sake of completeness. It is isolated rarely from sporadic cases of acute upper respiratory illness. Outbreaks are exceedingly rare. No vaccine has been prepared against it.

IMMUNIZING ANTIGEN

Influenza vaccine is a formalin-killed preparation of virus grown in the allantoic cavity of embryonated hens' eggs. This form of vaccine is more than 40 years old but various modifications have been introduced in preparation, designed to either increase the potency or to decrease the number of side-effects. The protein content of the vaccine has been reduced markedly and all modern vaccines are purified by zonal centrifugation or chromatography.

A recent modification has been the development of ether-split (hemagglutinin) vaccine. Experience with the effectiveness of such preparations has been limited but they considerably reduce the incidence of side-effects. The best evaluation of the potency and toxicity of these preparations was provided by the extensive field trials of monovalent swine vaccine and bivalent (Swine/A Victoria) vaccine in 1976. The split virus preparations produced fewer reactions but were also less potent than whole virus preparations.

Influenza vaccine is prepared from the most recent circulating strains. For example, the 1980–81 vaccine consisted of a trivalent preparation of A/Brazil/78 (H_1N_1), A Bangkok/79 (H_3N_2) and B/Singapore/79. That particular formulation contained 7 μg of hemagglutinin of each antigen in each 0.5 ml dose. Those 28 years of age or older needed only one dose. Because of lack of previous contact with H_1N_1 strains, those less than 28 years of age who had not received at least one dose of the 1978–79 or 1979–80 trivalent vaccine needed two doses of the 1980–81 vaccine; the remainder needed only one dose. That vaccine was available in whole version (whole virus) and subvirion (split virus) preparations. Only split virus vaccines were recommended for those less than 13 years of age because of the decreased side-effects of such preparations.

Each year, the Advisory Committee for Immunization Practices, with consultation of the Bureau of Biologics and the Redbook Committee of the American Academy of Pediatrics, considers the optimal formulation of influenza vaccine for the next year, both as to antigenic constituents and their concentrations and as to the recommended dose. These recommendations are made to pharmaceutical companies who then prepare the vaccines. The process from advice for formulation through vaccine preparation to delivery takes nearly a full year, so that antigenic drifts in the interim may severely limit the effectiveness of the vaccine. Major antigenic shifts (the emergence of a brand new variant) may result in abandonment of the old vaccine and a frantic effort to prepare a new one. In recent years of major shift, such effort has been unsuccessful, as it takes longer to prepare a potent new vaccine than it does for the new variant to spread, at least through the first wave.

The Armed Forces Epidemiologic Board makes separate recommendations for military use, usually the same in antigenic formulation, but often of increased dose of each antigen. For discussion of some new approaches to vaccine preparation for influenza viruses, see Chapter 25.

RATIONALE FOR VACCINE USE

Perhaps the best estimates of the effectiveness of recent influenza vaccines have been in the extensive trials in the military, primarily in young men. In 12 field studies performed over a 12-year period by the

Commission on Influenza, the protective effectiveness was 70 to 90%. Studies in civilians have given estimates of effectiveness of 60 to 80%. The difference could reflect the population difference but probably reflects the higher dose used in the military, often with more frequent side-effects. For example, in 1978 the H_1N_1 component was successful in preventing that variant of influenza in the military, but the vaccine distributed to civilians was notably ineffective.

The varying results reported in civilian trials reflect a number of problems. There is the question of antigenic similarity between the vaccine strains and the naturally occurring virus (how much antigenic drift has occurred?). Protection conferred by the vaccine wanes rather rapidly and the interval between immunization and the epidemic challenge is therefore critical. A conservative estimate is that vaccines are 75% effective for one year and approximately 50% effective for at least 18 months.

The dose of vaccine is another critical factor in effectiveness, and the problem that vaccine formulators face is to devise a protective dose that will not result in an unacceptable rate of side-effects. A final critical factor is the immune status of the recipient. Has priming by a previous infection or immunization with related influenza antigens occurred? It has been shown clearly in recent studies that the protective effect is limited to those not already immune who are vaccinated for the first time with the most recent strain. Revaccination with the same strain does not increase the degree of protection. Thus, when a new antigenic subtype first appears and a population is completely susceptible, a vaccine will have its maximum effect. However, the benefit is short-lived. As a strain undergoes antigenic drift, those previously protected from natural infection by vaccination will be at risk and cannot be effectively protected by further vaccination with the same strain.

The primary aim of vaccination with killed influenza vaccines (KIV) is prevention of mortality among those at high risk. Conditions predisposing to such risk include: (1) acquired or congenital heart diseases associated with altered circulatory dynamics, such as mitral stenosis, congestive heart failure, and pulmonary vascular overload; (2) any chronic disorder with compromised pulmonary function, such as chronic obstructive pulmonary disease, bronchiectasis, tuberculosis, severe asthma, cystic fibrosis, neuromuscular and orthopedic disorders with impaired ventilation, and residual pulmonary dysplasia following neonatal respiratory distress syndrome; (3) chronic renal disease with azotemia or the nephrotic syndrome; (4) diabetes mellitus and other metabolic diseases associated with an increased susceptibility to infection; (5) chronic severe anemia such as sickle cell disease; and (6) conditions that compromise the immune mechanism, including certain malignancies and immunosuppressive therapy.

The selection of the other segment of those at high risk—the aged—is made on the basis of studying the age-specific mortality of influenza, and immunization is, for that reason, recommended for those over age 65. There is debate as to whether healthy older persons are in fact at higher risk, but the excess mortality that is realized in epidemic influenza is greater than the frequency of the high-risk conditions listed in the foregoing, so that vaccination of all older persons is prudent and has been shown to reduce mortality in this general population.

With the introduction of a new variant, consideration should also be given to vaccinating those who provide essential community services, such as fire, police, military, and medical personnel.

In the 1918 and 1957 pandemics, an increased risk of maternal mortality from influenza in pregnant women was recorded. This has not been seen in other periods. The question of whether maternal influenza causes congenital malformations or leukemia in offspring is still unclear. Thus, at present, pregnant women should be considered for vaccination like all others. Killed vaccine is not contraindicated in pregnancy.

Current vaccine programs are not designed to affect the spread of influenza by use of vaccine, in contrast to the aim of vaccination against measles or polio, for example. There have been attempts to study the potential of immunizing school children, the initial focus of disease in epidemics. A theoretic model has shown that community attack rates should be reduced from 43% to 8% when 90% of school children are vaccinated. This theory has been tested in Tecumseh, Michigan, where approximately 10,000 (85%) of the school children were vaccinated. During the outbreak of Hong Kong (H_3N_2) influenza that followed vaccination with a vaccine containing that strain, there was a third as much illness in Tecumseh as in Adrian, a neighboring town which had no vaccine program. A month later, both communities had similar attack rates for influenza B, against which neither town had been vaccinated. Thus, even with this massive effort, a minimal effect was gained and there is no rationale for widespread use of the current KIV preparations in healthy children.

SIDE-EFFECTS OF AND ADVERSE REACTIONS TO VACCINATION

The major side-effects of influenza vaccination are fever, erythema, and tenderness at the site of immunization. Although side-effects can be due to extraneous materials such as endotoxin, they are also the result of reaction to killed influenza virus antigens. Side-effects from vaccination occur more frequently as the concentration of vaccine antigen increases and less frequently when the vaccinee has specific antibody to the vaccine viral antigens. These reactions begin 6 to 12 hours after vaccination and persist for 1 to 2 days.

Immediate responses, presumably allergic, such as flare and wheal, or respiratory expressions of hypersensitivity, are extremely rare. They are probably caused by allergy to vaccine constituents, most likely egg protein. A history of anaphylactic hypersensitivity to eggs (lip or tongue swelling, respiratory symptoms, or collapse) is a contraindication to vaccination. A useful rule is that if the patient cannot eat a whole egg without allergic symptoms developing, the vaccine is contraindicated.

Until 1976, only ten instances of neurologic complications following vaccination had been reported. The varying nature of symptoms (polyneuropathy, radiculopathy, encephalopathy) along with the lack of any recognizable pattern made such complications appear to be coincidental. After the swine influenza inoculation program of 1976, a careful assessment of illness and death following vaccination was made in the 42 million persons who were vaccinated. No illness or deaths in vaccine recipients were linked to vaccine with the exception of mild allergic or febrile reactions and a probable association with Guillain-Barre syndrome (GBS). The latter finding prompted a detailed inquiry into that association. For the ten weeks following vaccination, the excess risk was found to be approximately ten cases of GBS (5% fatality) for every million persons vaccinated—an incidence five to six times higher than that in unvaccinated persons. Those under 25 years of age had a lower relative risk than did others and also had a lower case-fatality rate.

Since that time, the CDC has continued a surveillance of GBS. Between January 1, 1978 and March 31, 1979, 1034 cases of GBS were reported to the CDC by members of the American Academy of Neurology. The syndrome is more common in men than in women, in whites than in blacks, and is most common in the 50 to 74 year age group. Two-thirds had antecedent illness (within eight weeks), 5% had undergone surgery, and only 3% had received a vaccination within eight weeks of illness onset. For the 1978–79 influenza vaccine, the relative risk of contracting GBS was 1.4 (compared with 6.2 relative risk for the same period for A/New Jersey [swine] influenza vaccine). Thus, it appears that besides the fact that there was intensive surveillance for the period of the swine influenza program, and besides the fact that there were so many vaccinated, there was an increased propensity for that vaccine to result in GBS. Nevertheless, GBS must remain a potential risk for recipients of KIV to be compared with the risk of influenza and its complications.

REFERENCES

Advisory Committee on Immunization Practices. Influenza vaccine 1980– 81. Morb Mort Week Rep 29:225, 1980

Center for Disease Control. Guillain Barre Syndrome Surveillance Report. January 1978– 79, October, 1980

Davenport FM: Influenza viruses. In Evans AD (ed): Viral Infections in Humans: Epidemiology and Control. New York, Plenum Press, 1976

Galasso GJ, Tyeryar FJ, Cate TR et al (eds): Clinical studies of influenza vaccines. J Infect Dis (Suppl) 136:S341– S746, 1977

Gregg MB, Bregman DJ, O'Brien RJ, Miller JD: Influenza related mortality. JAMA 239:115, 1978

Gregg MB, Hinman AR, Craven RB: The Russian flu: Its history and implications for this year's influenza season. JAMA 240:2260, 1978

Hoskins TW, Davies JR, Smith AJ et al: Assessment of inactivated influenza A vaccine after three outbreaks of influenza A at Christ's Hospital. Lancet 1:33, 1979

Kilbourne ED (ed): The Influenza Viruses and Influenza. New York, Academic Press, 1975

Kilbourne ED: The molecular epidemiology of influenza. J Infect Dis 127:478, 1973

Marks JS, Halpin TJ: Guillain Barre syndrome in recipients of A/New Jersey influenza vaccine. JAMA 243:2490, 1980

Masurel N, Marine W: Recycling of Asian and Hong Kong influenza virus. Am J Epidemiol 97:44, 1973

Monto AS, Davenport FM, Napier JA et al: Modification of an outbreak of influenza in Tecumseh, Michigan, by vaccination of school children. J Infect Dis 122:16, 1970

Neustadt RE, Fineberg HV: The Swine Flu Affair. US Department of Health, Education and Welfare, 1978

Osborn J (ed): History, Science and Politics. Influenza in America 1918– 1976. New York, Prodist, 1977

Schoenbaum SC, MacNeil BJ, Kavet J: The swine influenza decision. New Engl J Med 295:759, 1976

Stuart-Harris CH, Schild GC: Influenza; The Virus and the Disease. Littleton, MA, Publishing Sciences Group, 1976

17
Tuberculosis (BCG)

E. Russell Alexander

DISEASE

Tuberculosis in the United States is usually caused by respiratory infection with *Mycobacterium tuberculosis*. In the past, before pasteurization and control of bovine tuberculosis, the disease was acquired through ingestion of infected milk. For the great majority of those infected, primary infection is asymptomatic, and results only in conversion of the tuberculin skin test from negative to positive.

Tubercular lower respiratory disease may follow primary infection; dissemination of the organism is rare and most commonly results in miliary disease or meningitis. These severe forms of tuberculosis most commonly affect infants, the aged, and those who are malnourished or have other debilitating disease. The most common forms of tuberculosis now seen in the United States are secondary to reactivation or endogenous reinfection.

The steady and continuing decline of tuberculosis began before the turn of this century and is attributable to changes in our standard of living; decreased crowding, improved nutrition, and generally improved hygiene have had a significant impact in reducing transmission and disease. However, a further incremental decrease is attributable to isolation and nonspecific treatment and to specific antibiotic and chemotherapeutic treatment of sputum-positive cases. In recent years, the success of tuberculosis control in this country has been partially related to "prophylaxis" with isoniazid, the prophylaxis meaning treatment of tuberculin-positive persons in order to prevent disease. Isoniazid treatment has been successful and is the primary control method in use in the United States. Bacille Calmette-Guerin (BCG) vaccine is rarely used; it is limited to special circumstances which will be detailed later.

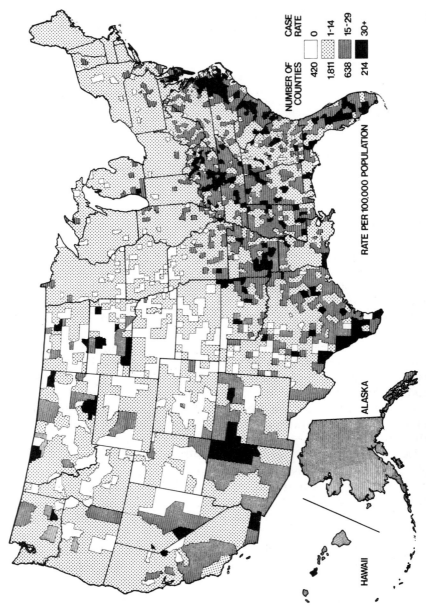

CASE RATE

NUMBER OF COUNTIES	CASE RATE
420	0
1,811	1–14
638	15–29
214	30+

RATE PER 100,000 POPULATION

ALASKA

HAWAII

Fig. 17-1. Tuberculosis: reported average cases per 100,000 population by county, United States, 1976–1978 (Center for Disease Control. Morb Mort Week Rep, 28:54, 1980 [Annual Summary 1979])

In 1980, there were 27,983 reported cases of tuberculosis in the United States (12.4 per 100,000 population). In the last year for which mortality statistics are available (1977), there were 30,000 cases and 3,000 deaths for rates of 13.9 and 1.4/100,000 respectively. In the decade between 1967 and 1977, cases and deaths declined 40% and 60%, respectively (Fig. 17-1). The decrease for 1979–80 is only 1.6%. The prevalence of infection is measured by the prevalence of positive tuberculin skin tests. For children, the percentage at school entrance is 0.2% and in adolescence, 0.7%. The annual infection rate is estimated to be 0.03%. To a large extent, tuberculosis is a disease of certain population segments. It is concentrated in impoverished persons with inadequate health care, the prevalence still being higher in blacks and in American Indians (Figs. 17-1 and 17-2). The prevalence is also particularly high in immigrants from other countries, currently Indochina refugees in particular.

The great majority of cases of recurrence are among adult patients, with men more often affected than women (Fig. 17-2). Most often, careful search for sources will reveal unrecognized or untreated sputum-positive cases.

IMMUNIZING ANTIGEN

The bacillus of Calmette and Guerin was originally derived from a virulent strain of *Mycobacterium bovis*, attenuated by 231 serial passages over 13 years. Earlier attempts by Koch and others to treat tuberculosis with injections of killed bacilli ended disastrously with illness and, in some, death. The BCG vaccine was first used orally in infants in 1921. An accident occurred in Lubeck, Germany, in the 1930s and resulted in virulent mycobacteria being inoculated instead of an attenuated strain, and 72 infants so inoculated died.

Following this, a series of controlled trials were conducted in the United States, then in Puerto Rico, England and India during the period between 1935 and 1955. The vaccine was judged to be reasonably safe but the protective effectiveness varied from 10% to 80%; three trials showed excellent protection; two, mediocre protection; and two, poor protection. Results of a number of smaller, less well-controlled studies were similarly disparate.

Three hypotheses have been suggested to explain these results. The first is that in areas where atypical mycobacteria are prevalent, such as the southeastern United States, BCG vaccine can only be expected to supplement existing cross-immunity. Although such a phenomenon may contribute to the disparities, it can by no means be the sole explanation. The second hypothesis is that, because greatest effectiveness had been shown in areas of greatest prevalence, superinfection with

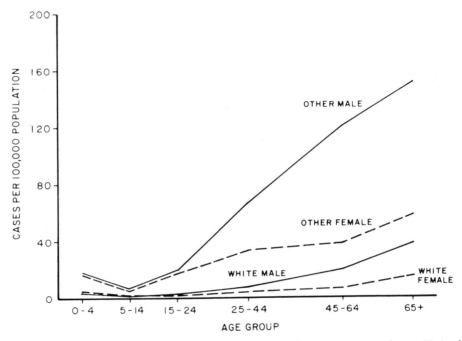

Fig. 17-2. Tuberculosis: reported case rates by race, sex, and age, United States, 1979 (Center for Disease Control. Morb Mort Week Rep, 28:54, 1980 [Annual Summary 1979])

virulent tubercle bacilli may be necessary in order to attain adequate protection from BCG. This hypothesis has not been disproven and may be valid. A third hypothesis is that BCG vaccines are not identical. For example, in the seven large controlled trials mentioned, five different strains of BCG were used, prepared in five different laboratories. Although the original attenuated strain prepared at the Pasteur Institute was the progenitor of all of them, it was distributed to hundreds of laboratories in many countries and maintained by serial subculture in each of them. Therefore, many different "daughter" BCG strains exist that differ in gross morphology, growth characteristics, biochemical activity, sensitivity, potency, and animal virulence. In the last two decades, most laboratories have adopted a seed lot system, and lyophilization of production strains tends to minimize genetic variation.

Nevertheless, existing BCG vaccines vary in immunogenicity, effectiveness, and reactogenicity. Current vaccines all differ from those used in the field trials previously mentioned. There have been further modifications in methods of preparation and preservation. The effectiveness of current vaccines has not been demonstrated directly and can only be inferred. Production standards for BCG vaccines in the United States specify that they be freeze-dried and that they contain live bacteria from a documented BCG strain with specified characteristics of safety and potency. All strains must be capable of inducing tuberculin sensitivity in guinea pigs and humans, despite the fact that the relationship between sensitivity and immunity has not been proven.

Because of the conflicting results from prior trials, a large controlled field trial of flawless design was conducted in Madras, India, with the collaboration of the Indian Council of Medical Research, the World Health Organization (WHO), and the United States Public Health Service, and involved 260,000 participants. Freeze-dried vaccines prepared in two laboratories were chosen because they were among the most potent in use in recent years. The results so far have been negative; slightly more tuberculosis cases have appeared in vaccinated than in equal-sized placebo control groups. Not only the design, but also the conduct and analysis of the trial were excellent. The WHO has reviewed the results and cannot fault the methods or conclusions. There appear to be no ready explanations for this result. The questions about BCG use persist. Protection is unpredictable and is at best less than we demand for most vaccines. For example, the comparable Medical Research Council statistics in the United Kingdom suggest 70% protection over 10 years.

As a result of the India trial, the WHO has authorized similarly designed studies in selected populations, including children, to determine whether any BCG effectiveness is demonstrable.

IMMUNITY TO TUBERCULOSIS

The exact role of immune responses to *M. tuberculosis* in recovery from infection and maintenance of the asymptomatic state is uncertain. Cell-mediated immunity (CMI), manifested by both *in vitro* and *in vivo* (tuberculin sensitivity) and *in vitro* (lymphocyte stimulation) responses, appears to be most critical. However, CMI response *in vivo* also serves as part of the pathogenesis of clinical disease and in reactivation. Differentiating the immune from the pathogenetic role has been difficult.

Complicating this assessment has been the MOTT organisms (so-called mycobacteria other than tuberculosis or atypical mycobacteria) existing in various parts of the world. Tuberculin sensitivity to these organisms develops and its role in immunity to *M. tuberculosis* is also unclear.

Most likely, positive tuberculin CMI is linked to the lymphocyte's capacity to limit the spread of organisms in primary infections and to keep viable organisms contained within inflammatory foci. Subtle changes in the level of CMI may account for reactivation or autoinfection. Age, stress, nutrition, medications, and certain diseases appear to influence susceptibility as does an ill-defined genetic predisposition.

RATIONALE FOR USE

In the United States, the methods of case detection, chemotherapy, and preventive treatment remain the cornerstones of a very effective control program. The BCG vaccine is a potentially useful adjunct in infrequent instances in which persons with reported exposure to infective cases cannot or will not accept the usual treatment. This use is based on the assumption that BCG does confer some protection. Potential recipients include infants who are tuberculin-skin-test-negative with persistent exposure to untreated or inadequately treated persons in the household who are sputum-positive. Another example is those in population groups in which an excessive rate of new infections persists and in which the usual case detection treatment and preventive methods cannot be used, such as when persons are outside the reach of health-care systems. A third example is tuberculin-negative persons who plan to live in areas of high endemicity who cannot avail themselves of the usual surveillance and control methods. A fourth group which has been considered for BCG in the past, health workers with high exposure, is not considered any longer. Instead, repeated skin test evaluation is recommended and is far more effective in control.

One potential deficit of BCG administration is the loss of skin test conversion as an index of newly acquired infection. Some experts decry the use of BCG for this reason.

SCHEDULING AND ADMINISTRATION

Vaccine recipients should be negative to tuberculin skin testing to five tuberculin units of tuberculin purified protein derivative (PPD). Dosage is indicated by the manufacturer in the package labeling. Half the dose (usually 0.1 ml) should be given to infants less than 1 month of age. If the indications for vaccination persist, these infants should be given additional full doses after their first birthdays. Injections are given intradermally, usually over the deltoid or triceps muscle, as superficially as possible. Those who receive BCG should have tuberculin tests two to three months later and, if negative, should be revaccinated. Tuberculin conversion as a result of BCG can persist for 4 years or more, particularly if the individual has been asymptomatically infected with *M. tuberculosis* under cover of BCG-provided partial immunity.

SIDE-EFFECTS AND ADVERSE REACTIONS

Adverse reactions include severe or prolonged ulceration or suppurative abscesses at the vaccination site, lymphadenitis, and, more rarely, osteomyelitis, lupoid reactions, disseminated BCG infection, and death. As with effectiveness data, reports of adverse reactions vary considerably, reflecting differences in vaccines and recipients. Most of the adverse reactions occur more commonly in the neonate. Thus, the frequency of ulceration and lymphadenitis ranges from 1% to 10%.

Regional lymphadenitis is a major side-effect, because it may not be recognized as being linked with BCG. Removal of the nodes is not indicated. Histologic examination may confuse the inflammatory changes seen with other infectious or malignant processes.

Osteomyelitis generally occurs in one per million recipients (although the rate has been reported to be as high as five per 100,000 in newborns). Disseminated BCG infection and death are extremely rare (less than one per million vaccinees) and are believed to occur exclusively in children with impaired immune responses, especially those with T-cell or CMI deficiencies.

PRECAUTIONS AND CONTRAINDICATIONS

Persons who should not be given BCG include those with impaired immune responses such as occur with congenital immunodeficiency, leukemia, lymphoma, or generalized malignancy and those with immunosuppression by steroids, aklylating agents, antimetabolites or radiation.

Although BCG has not been shown to be harmful to the fetus or the pregnant mother, vaccination in pregnancy should be avoided if possible.

SPECIAL NOTE—TUBERCULIN TESTING

The tuberculin test is a valuable case-finding tool. In ordinary pediatric practice, it is recommended that a reliable and reproducible method be used for tuberculin skin testing of patients at 12 months of age and yearly or every two years thereafter. This recommendation is based upon the value of detecting asymptomatic converters and providing isoniazid prophylaxis to prevent disease, especially tuberculous meningitis.

Some public health experts, including those at the CDC, suggest that tuberculin testing be eliminated if the prevalence of positive reactors falls below 1% in any given population. Current prevalence rates in many parts of the United States are well below this level. The Academy of Pediatrics still maintains that detection of any cases in ordinary practice is worthwhile, given the low cost and minimal risk of tuberculin testing. This body does recognize that, in some circumstances, the practitioner may wish to either alter the frequency of testing (much longer intervals between tests) or to abandon it entirely.

Screening tests for tuberculin sensitivity have replaced the standard 5TU intradermal method (Mantoux test) in many areas. Recently, questions have been raised concerning the reliability of these procedures. The FDA is conducting a comparison of commonly used screening test results with the Mantoux reactions. Until the results of this field trial are known, the practitioner should either: (1) use only Mantoux testing at the 5TU level (intermediate strength PPD); or (2) use the screening test with scrupulous attention to the manufacturer's recommendations for both drug administration and interpretation of results.

All tuberculin tests are best read and interpreted by a trained professional. The common practice of having parents read the test can be effective if care is taken to give proper instructions, and if a convenient and simple method for recording results and reporting them, such as a printed, stamped postal card, is made available.

REFERENCES

Advisory Committee on Immunization Practices. BCG vaccine. Morb Mort Week Rep 28:241, 1979

Comstock GW: Frost revisited: The modern epidemiology of tuberculosis. Am J Epidemiol 101:363, 1975

Dash LA, Comstock GW, Glynn JPG: Isoniazid prevention retrospect and prospect. Am Rev Respir Dis 121:1039, 1980

Eickhoff TC: The current status of BCG immunization against tuberculosis. Ann Rev Med 28:411, 1977

Glassroth J, Robins AG, Snider DE Jr: Tuberculosis in the 1980's. New Engl J Med 302:1441, 1980

Hart PDA, Sutherland I: BCG and vole bacillus vaccines in the prevention of tuberculosis in adolescence and early life. Final report to the Medical Research Council. Br Med J 2:293, 1977

Leff A, Geppert EF: Public health and preventive aspects of pulmonary tuberculosis— infectiousness, epidemiology, risk factors, classification and preventive therapy. Arch Intern Med 139:1405, 1979

Tendam HG, Hitze KL: Does BCG vaccination protect the newborn and young infants? Bull WHO 58:37, 1980

Tuberculosis Prevention Trial Madras. Trial of BCG vaccines in South India for tuberculosis prevention. Ind J Med Res 70:349, 1979

18

Yellow Fever

C. George Ray

DISEASE

While endemic in areas of Africa and Central and South America, yellow fever is of limited significance in the United States. In the 19th century, seaports such as Philadelphia, New York, and New Orleans were affected by epidemics. The last major outbreak in the United States was in New Orleans in 1905. Nevertheless, the risk of infection and disease still exists for travelers to and from endemic areas, and the proximity of some of these areas to the United States along with the existence of the mosquito vector (*Aedes aegypti*) within our borders suggest the remote possibility of reintroduction of the problem (Figs. 18-1 and 18-2).

The incubation period for yellow fever ranges from 3 to 14 days and is followed by the sudden onset of fever, nausea, vomiting, headache, and myalgia. This sometimes progresses to jaundice and may be accompanied by hepatic and renal failure. Mortality rates range from 5% in endemic situations to as much as 40% in certain age groups during epidemics. If the patient survives the acute infection, recovery is usually complete and without sequelae.

The major method of control is aimed at reducing the insect vector. Immunization does play an important role in protection and is strongly recommended (or sometimes required) for those traveling to areas of known virus activity. In order to determine whether vaccination is necessary, travelers should contact their local health departments for advice.

Two forms of yellow fever—urban and jungle—are distinguishable epidemiologically, but not clinically. Urban yellow fever is transmitted from person to person via *Aedes aegypti* mosquitos and can be best eradicated by insect control programs.

Jungle yellow fever has a more complex cycle of transmission, involv-

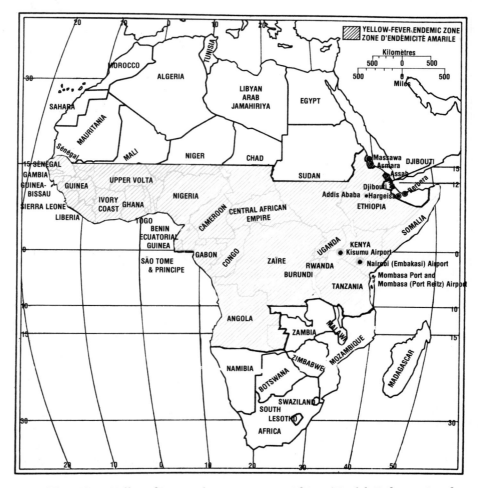

Fig. 18-1. Yellow fever endemic zones in Africa (Health Information for International Travel. Atlanta, Center for Disease Control, 1980)

ing animals such as monkeys and a variety of insect vectors. Humans are infected incidentally if they intrude into this cycle. The only effective means of preventing jungle fever is immunization.

IMMUNIZING ANTIGEN

Two strains of yellow fever vaccine are approved by the World Health Organization (WHO): the Dakar (or French neurotropic) strain and the 17D strain. Both are live, attenuated virus vaccines. The Dakar strain is not used in the United States; it has been associated with a high

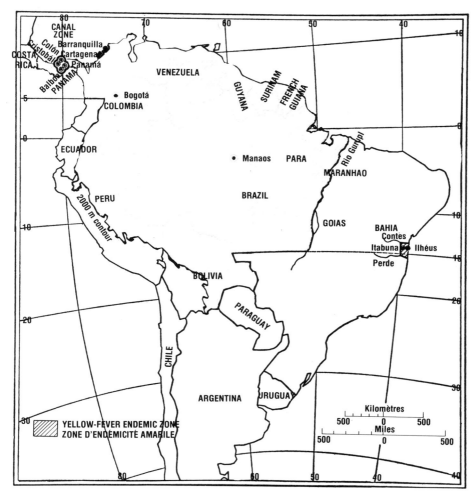

Fig. 18-2. Yellow fever endemic zones in the Americas (Health Information for Travel. Atlanta, Center for Disease Control, 1980)

incidence of encephalitis reactions (0.5%), especially among children less than 14 years of age.

The 17D vaccine was derived from the Asibi strain of virus which was maintained for 18 subcultures in embryonic mouse tissue and for 218 subcultures in chick embryo cultures. It is supplied as a freeze-dried supernate of centrifuged chick embryo homogenate. It must be administered within an hour of being reconstituted and the remainder must be discarded. The vaccine can *only* be obtained and administered at a yellow fever vaccination center. Travelers should be advised to call their local health departments for information on centers in their area.

RATIONALE FOR ACTIVE IMMUNIZATION

Only persons at least 6 months old who are traveling to infected areas where certificates of vaccination are required for entry or where vaccination is strongly recommended are considered candidates for immunization. The only exception would be workers in laboratories that might conduct research with the virus.

IMMUNITY

It has been shown that neutralizing and hemagglutination-inhibition antibodies persist in humans for at least 16 to 19 years after a single dose of 17D vaccine. The antibody titers achieved appear to correlate well with protective immunity.

SCHEDULING OF IMMUNIZATION

A single subcutaneous injection of 0.5 ml of reconstituted vaccine is used for both adults and children. If booster doses are needed, they need not be given more often than once every ten years, in the same volume.

Special Circumstances. In the nonimmune host, viremia associated with the induction of circulating interferon develops three to nine days after immunization. If circumstances dictate that other live-virus vaccines such as vaccinia or measles are also required for travel, it is recommended that these be given 28 days apart from the yellow fever vaccine in order to avoid interference. This was a major consideration when smallpox vaccine was also frequently required; however, the need for smallpox immunization has been significantly diminished and may become nonexistent in the next several years. Furthermore, it has been shown in volunteer studies that careful spacing of smallpox and yellow fever vaccines may not be essential.

When killed vaccines, such as cholera, are given simultaneously with yellow fever vaccine, there is some evidence that immune responses to both vaccines may be reduced (see Chap. 22).

SIDE-EFFECTS AND ADVERSE REACTIONS TO IMMUNIZATION

The 17D vaccine is minimally reactogenic. Five percent to 10% of vaccinees will have mild headache, myalgia, low-grade fever, or other minor symptoms five to ten days after vaccination, but less than 0.2%

curtail regular activities. Only two cases of encephalitis have been reported to be associated with the vaccine in the United States, despite the fact that more than 34 million doses have been administered.

SPECIFIC PRECAUTIONS

Pregnancy. There is no evidence that yellow fever vaccine has an adverse effect on the pregnant woman or her developing fetus; however, it is considered prudent to avoid administering any live vaccine in this situation, if at all possible. If a woman must travel to an endemic area while pregnant, vaccination is recommended if the risk of acquiring yellow fever is considered to be high compared to the theoretic risk associated with the vaccine.

Altered Immune States. Primary or acquired immunodeficiency states are all contraindicatory to yellow fever immunization.

Infants Less Than 6 Months of Age. The international and United States recommendations exclude infants less than six months of age. The primary reasons for this exclusion relate to little experience with routine vaccination in this age group, and the possibility that young infants may be relatively immunodeficient in their ability to respond appropriately with an adequate antibody response. In addition, there is considered to be a higher (but undefined) risk of postvaccination encephalitis in infancy.

Hypersensitivity. The vaccine is produced in chick embryo cell cultures and should not be given to persons known to be egg-sensitive. Also, the vaccine contains traces of antibiotics and may pose a risk to persons sensitive to these.

If international travel regulations mandate a validated certificate of immunization for a patient who is at risk for a severe hypersensitivity reaction, efforts should be made to obtain a waiver. The following approach has been suggested by the Public Health Service Advisory Committee on Immunization Practices:

> A physician's letter clearly stating the contraindication to vaccination has been acceptable to some governments. (Ideally, it should be written on the letterhead stationery and bear the stamp used by health departments and official immunization centers to validate international certificates of vaccination.) Under these conditions it is also useful for the traveler to obtain specific and authoritative advice from the country or countries he or she plans to visit. Their embassies or consulates may be contacted. Subsequent waiver of requirements should be documented by appropriate letters.

REFERENCES

Recommendation of Public Health Service Advisory Committee on Immunization Practices. Morb Mort Week Rep 27:268–270, 1978

Robbins FC, Mahmoud AA, Warren KS: Algorithms in the diagnosis and management of exotic diseases. XIX. Major tropical viral infections: smallpox, yellow fever, and lassa fever. J Infect Dis 135:341–346, 1977

Rosenzweig EC, Babione RW, Wisseman CL Jr: Immunological studies with group B arthropod-borne viruses. IV. Persistence of yellow fever antibodies following vaccination with 17D strain yellow fever vaccine. Am J Trop Med Hyg 12:230–235, 1963

Tauraso NM, Myers MG, Nau EV et al: Effect of interval between inoculation of live smallpox and yellow fever vaccines on antigenicity in man. J Infect Dis 126:362–371, 1972

19

Typhoid Fever (Salmonella Septicemia)

C. George Ray

DISEASE

Salmonella typhi (formerly *Salmonella typhosa*) is the major cause of the septicemic diseases known as typhoid fever. Other salmonella species, including *S. choleraesuis* and *S. enteritidis* (includes more than 1700 serotypes as well as the previously named paratyphoid A, B, and C serotypes) are also capable of producing typhoidlike diseases but are generally less often implicated. The *S. enteritidis* serotypes are primarily causes of gastroenteritis, which will not be considered in this chapter.

The average incubation period of typhoid fever after oral exposure is 7.5 days, with a range of 3 to 33 days. Typically, there is a gradual onset, with fever, headache, myalgia, anorexia, and dry cough. Later in the illness, abdominal pain and tenderness, bloody stools, and "rose spots" may develop. Children will also frequently experience vomiting and diarrhea and the leukopenia that is often observed in adult patients may not develop. The untreated disease lasts 3 to 4 weeks. In the preantibiotic era, mortality rates were estimated to be 12% to 16%; with specific therapy, present-day mortality is less than 1%. However, 1% to 3% of infected persons who recover become chronic carriers and may shed the organism in their feces for years afterward.

In the United States, the annual incidence of typhoid fever has decreased to less than 400 reported cases annually and a downward trend continues. Nearly half of these cases have been acquired outside the United States.

IMMUNIZING ANTIGEN

Several different types of typhoid vaccines have been used in the past. Those containing paratyphoid A and B as well as typhoid antigens (TAB) have not been shown to be advantageous and do increase the risk of vaccine reactions—these should *not* be used.

The preferred vaccine is a saline suspension of acetone-killed *S. typhi*. This should not be given intradermally.

RATIONALE FOR ACTIVE IMMUNIZATION

Routine typhoid immunization is not recommended in the United States. Selective immunization is indicated only when (1) there will be close household-type contact with documented typhoid carriers, or (2) there will be travel to high-risk areas where food and water sanitation is poor and typhoid fever is known to exist.

Typhoid vaccine has not been shown to be effective in controlling common-source outbreaks in the United States. In addition, there is no value in using the vaccine for victims of natural disasters such as floods or for persons attending summer camps.

IMMUNITY

Even immunity derived from naturally acquired infections is imperfect, although reinfection is unusual. Also, there is no correlation between the occurrence of relapse of disease and the levels of circulating antibody titers to the O, H, or Vi antigens of the typhoid bacillus. With these facts in mind, it is not too surprising that vaccine-induced immunity is somewhat unpredictable and of uncertain duration. Patients should be informed of these uncertainties lest they rely too much on vaccine-induced protection and overlook the need to exercise care in hygienic practices and in selection of foods and drinks.

Vaccine-induced immunity can be readily overcome with oral challenge doses of 10^7 or more live *S. typhi* organisms in human volunteers. At challenge levels of 10^5 organisms, protective efficacy has been shown to be 67%, and is probably greater (from 70% to 90%) at even lower doses which may be encountered in a natural setting. The duration of protection is uncertain.

Results of experimental trials using oral immunization with either live attenuated mutant strains of *S. typhi* or killed bacteria are varied. Such vaccines have not been released for general use.

SCHEDULING OF IMMUNIZATION

Primary Immunization. Adult patients and children 10 years of age and older should be given two 0.5 ml doses subcutaneously, the second dose at least 4 weeks after the first. Children less than 10 years of age should be given two 0.25 ml doses subcutaneously, the doses again separated by 4 weeks or more.

Booster Immunization. If continued exposure is expected, booster doses are given at three-year intervals or more, depending on whether exposure is continuous or intermittent. Persons 10 years of age and older should receive 0.5 ml subcutaneously and those under 10 years should receive 0.25 ml subcutaneously.

Intradermal boosters of 0.1 ml for all ages are alternatively recommended because they generally produce fewer reactions. If this route is employed, acetone-killed vaccine should *not* be used; a non-acetone-killed vaccine is available for this purpose.

SIDE-EFFECTS AND ADVERSE REACTIONS

The majority of typhoid vaccine recipients will experience local reactions with varying discomfort and occasionally erythema, tenderness, and swelling at the site of injection for 1 to 2 days afterward. This may be accompanied by fever, malaise, and headache. Febrile reactions are particularly common in children and antipyretic treatment may be indicated. Transient or regional lymphadenopathy may also occur.

SPECIFIC PRECAUTIONS

It is generally wise to withhold use of the vaccine in pregnancy, even though there are no known adverse side-effects in this situation.

If patients who have experienced severe reactions to prior typhoid immunization need subsequent doses, including boosters, they should be given in reduced amounts. Intradermal boosters of the non-acetone-killed vaccine are particularly useful in such situations.

REFERENCES

Butler T, Mahmoud AAF, Warren KS: Algorithms in the diagnosis and management of exotic diseases: XXIII. Typhoid fever. J Infect Dis 135:1017–1020, 1977
Colon AR, Gross DR, Tamer MA: Typhoid fever in children. Pediatrics 56:606–609, 1975

Hornick RB, Greisman SE, Woodward TE et al: Typhoid fever: Pathogenesis and immunologic control. New Engl J Med 283:686– 691, 739, 746, 1970
Hornick RB, Woodward TE, McCrumb FR et al: Typhoid fever vaccine—yes or no? Med Clin North Am 51:617– 623, 1967
Recommendations of the Public Health Service Advisory Committee on Immunization Practices. Morb Mort Week Rep 27:231– 233, 1978

20

Pneumococcal
Infections

H. Robert Harrison

DISEASE

Although the mortality rates of pneumococcal infections have decreased markedly since the introduction of effective antibiotics, attack rates are still appreciable and have probably not declined at all. Further, penicillin-resistant strains have recently been identified in clinical infections.

Pneumococcal pneumonia is still the most common community-acquired bacterial pneumonia in all age groups. Although epidemics in closed populations have been rare since 1950, it is estimated that there are still 500,000 cases annually in this country. Even with early and appropriate antibiotic therapy, the case fatality rate may be as high as 10% to 15% and reaches 28% for those over 50 years old or with chronic systemic illness.

Pneumococcal meningitis occurs in approximately 1.5 to 2.5 per 100,000 population per year. Half these patients are infants or children. Of the three major pediatric meningitides (*Haemophilus influenzae, Neisseria meningitidis, Streptococcus pneumoniae*), pneumococcal meningitis is the most serious in terms of permanent neurologic sequelae and mortality, even with early, appropriate therapy.

Occult pneumococcal bacteremia is predominantly a pediatric illness, presenting predominantly in infants between 6 and 24 months of age with acute fever without obvious source. Many of these infants will have an underlying otitis media or pneumonia and as many as 10% of them will subsequently have pneumococcal meningitis. Occult bacteremia can also occur, at lesser rates, throughout childhood.

Pneumococcal disease of all types is very common in persons with anatomic or functional asplenia, congenital heart disease with asplenia-polysplenia, and in those with surgical splenectomy.

In addition, pneumococcal infections are a serious problem in some children with malignancies, in those on immunosuppressive or antineoplastic therapy, and in those with nephrotic syndrome, chronic liver disease, or antibody immunodeficiencies, whether congenital or acquired.

There are currently 83 identified capsular serotypes of *Streptococcus pneumoniae* (pneumococcus). However, certain types are more likely to cause human disease than are others. In a recent review of 293 pneumococcal isolates from bacteremic pediatric patients, only 27 different serotypes were identified. Furthermore, 11 of these caused 90% of the illness in all disease categories (pneumonia, meningitis, localized infections, bacteremia); none of the other 16 types accounted for more than 1% of the isolates. The most common types, 6, 14, and 19, in the Danish nomenclature, accounting for 45% of isolates in this study, have always been more commonly found in children than adults. The next three serotypes, 9, 18, and 23, accounted for 27% of isolates, and the remaining four, 3, 4, 7, and 8, have remained common in adult disease.

A second pediatric study of 101 isolates over a five year period identified 22 serotypes as major causes of disease. Of these, 12 capsular types (18, 19, 7, 23, 6, 1, 4, 14, 9, 3, 12, and 8 in order of decreasing prevalence) accounted for 91% of all illnesses. Thus, two separate surveys have shown a preponderance of a small group of serotypes in pediatric pneumococcal infection. A recent cross-sectional survey of 573 pneumococcal isolates sent to the Center for Disease Control (CDC) during a one year period (May 1978 to May 1979) showed the most common types in pediatric patients (those under 10 years old) to be 14, 19, 18, 6, and 23, and the most common types in adult patients (those more than 10 years old) to be 4, 3, 7, 23, and 8.

The relative paucity of specific serotypes producing serious disease suggests the possibility of control by immunization. Just prior to the advent of sulfonamides and the penicillins, there was increasing investigation and interest in vaccine development. With antimicrobial availability, these efforts diminished and have only recently been revised.

It has become clear over the last 30 years that antibiotics alone are not the sole answer to control of pneumococcal disease. Neither incidence rates nor case-to-fatality ratios in high-risk groups have changed appreciably during the antibiotic era. In addition, antibiotic-resistant strains have emerged among disease-producing pneumococci. There have been reports of a multiply-resistant pneumococci from South Africa as well as a highly penicillin-resistant strain from Minnesota. Furthermore, the CDC has observed relative penicillin resistance (MIC 0.1 to 0.5 μg/ml) in 15% of recent disease-producing isolates.

Armed with such data, investigators and clinicians have sought an effective and safe method for active immunization against pneumococci.

PRINCIPLES OF IMMUNITY

The pneumococcus is pathogenic by virtue of a polysaccharide capsule that renders it resistant to phagocytosis and subsequent destruction. Effective defense against and recovery from pneumococcal infection depends upon two components of the humoral immune system, antibody production and opsonization, for efficient phagocytosis by polymorphonuclear leukocytes. Antibody produced by B cells is directed against components of the bacterial polysaccharide capsule and provides some opsonic activity. However, both antibody and complement are needed for maximum antibody-enhanced phagocytosis of pneumococci. Immunity is type-specific with only a small degree of overlap among closely related strains and is of long duration. In general, the type-specific antibody is ineffective against nonrelated invading strains. This latter principle was responsible for the use of type-specific antiserum in the treatment of pneumococcal disease in the preantibiotic era, and it has been a continuing stimulus for vaccine development. Recent evidence also suggests that the pre-immunization serum IgG-2 concentration is strongly correlated with the ability to produce antibody.

PNEUMOCOCCAL VACCINE

Immunization has been a strategy in combating pneumococcal disease for most of this century. Trials using vaccines prepared from whole organisms were begun in South Africa in 1911. Capsular polysaccharide was discovered to be the immunogenic bacterial component in 1930. Purified capsular vaccine containing 50 μg of each of four type-specific preparations prevented pneumococcal pneumonia caused by those types in clinical trials in 1945. Protection coincided with the development of type-specific antibodies, which proved to be long-lasting. A hexavalent vaccine similar to that currently available was licensed and produced in the United States from 1945 to 1947. However, the introduction and usefulness of effective antibiotics against the pneumococcus resulted in diminished interest in, and use of, the vaccine and it was withdrawn.

Significant mortality from pneumococcal disease continued despite the availability of effective treatment. The emergence of resistant strains and continued morbidity led to a revival of interest in pneumococcal vaccine. Redevelopment began in 1967 under the auspices of the National Institute of Allergy and Infectious Diseases and was largely due to the efforts of Robert Austrian, one of the pioneers in pneumococcal research. Each 0.5 ml dose of the 14-valent polysaccharide vaccine now available contains 50 μg of purified capsular polysaccharide for each of the 14 serotypes (American types 1, 2, 3, 4, 6, 8, 9, 12, 14, 19, 23, 25, 51, and 56) reported to cause approximately 80% of the serious pneumococcal disease in the United States at the time of vaccine development. The carrier is isotonic saline solution, containing 0.25% phenol as a preservative.

VACCINE EFFECTIVENESS

There is currently a great deal of controversy over the effectiveness of pneumococcal vaccine, both in adult patients and in children, and it is expected to continue. The initial experience with adult patients was very favorable; controlled field trials on almost 28,000 adult patients both inside the United States and abroad have shown the vaccine to be highly effective in preventing pneumonia and bacteremia due to the capsular types included in the vaccine. Some conflicting data, however, have since emerged.

First, two separate studies have shown that 62% to 70% of isolates, rather than the expected 80%, are types represented in the vaccine. Second, in another investigation, which analyzed pneumococcal infections in persons vaccinated because of high risk for disease, the proportion of vaccine serotypes isolated from these patients was suprisingly similar to that from a group of unvaccinated normal persons. Furthermore, the estimated effectiveness was lowest in children 2 to 10 years old and in persons with pre-existing disease thought to predispose them to pneumococcal infection (0%), and highest in those over 10 years old (60%).

The resolution of this controversy may lie in both the variability of the immune response to the different vaccine serotypes and in the distinction between antibody titer and clinical effectiveness. Certain vaccine serotypes are "stronger" immunogens (American types 3, 4, 8, 9, and 23) than others (1, 6, 12, 14, 19, 51, and 56), inducing a stronger antibody response and at a younger age. Consequently, the vaccine may provide less overall protection against the weaker disease-producing serotypes. Also, clinical effectiveness depends upon factors other than antibody titer, such as serum IgG-2 level and complement activity. Thus, there may be both healthy and immunocompromised vaccinated persons with reasonable antibody responses who are still at risk for infection with vaccine strains.

Resolving these questions will depend upon further accumulation of data. To date, results of pediatric studies indicate that those less than 2 years old exhibit unsatisfactory serologic responses to a single dose of vaccine. Booster doses have no demonstrable effect on adult patients, and their effect on children is unknown. In a study of two small groups of children over 2 years old with sickle cell anemia and with splenectomy, the incidence of bacteremic pneumococcal disease seemed to be reduced significantly after immunization with a single dose of an 8-valent vaccine; the effect persisted during 2 years of continued observation.

In addition to its use in preventing serious pneumococcal disease, there is a great deal of interest in vaccination for preventing pneumococcal otitis media in children. Preliminary results of studies of small numbers of patients suggest that the vaccine may reduce the number of episodes of otitis during the first two years of life, despite the variable and unpredictable immune response. A great deal of work remains to be done before we can accurately evaluate the potential contribution of a pneumococcal vaccine in preventing pediatric otitis media, and the vaccine is not currently recommended for this purpose.

SCHEDULES OF IMMUNIZATION

The data currently available permit tentative recommendations. There is currently no indication for using the vaccine in children under 2 years of age, or for using it as a routine vaccination in healthy children regardless of age. The vaccine is recommended, however, in children over 2 years of age who are at risk for severe or life-threatening pneumococcal disease. Such children include those with sickle cell anemia and those postsplenectomy for other reasons. Children with Hodgkin's disease and perhaps other malignancies should be immunized prior to splenectomy or treatment since both of these interventions impair the host antibody and opsonic responses to vaccination. Children with nephrotic syndrome and those with antibody immunodeficiencies should be considered candidates for inoculation.

In all cases, a single 0.5 ml dose given subcutaneously or intramuscularly is recommended. This recommendation may change as experience in vaccinating children continues.

There is continuing controversy over the use of pneumococcal vaccine in children with chronic cardiac or respiratory disease including cystic fibrosis. It is currently felt that these conditions do not mandate immunization and use of vaccine is not recommended.

Theoretically, limited use of pneumococcal vaccine may be helpful in controlling outbreaks of pneumococcal disease in closed populations or in controlling geographically localized outbreaks in the community (very rare). However, there are no recommendations for use in these situations and the vaccine should probably not be used until its effectiveness has been demonstrated.

The majority of adult patients respond to vaccination with several-fold rises of type-specific antibody titers, which remain elevated for several years. Mass immunization of healthy adults is *not* recommended. Adult patients who should be immunized include those at high risk for pneumonococcal disease such as diabetics, those on immunosuppressive or antineoplastic therapy, those with functional or anatomic asplenia, and those with cardiorespiratory and renal impairments. In addition, those at high risk for influenza complications such as bacterial pneumonia should be vaccinated. Because both the risk of and the case-to-fatality ratio from pneumococcal disease increase with age, the benefits of vaccination are expected to increase as patients become older.

Booster doses of vaccine are currently considered unnecessary. In fact, some adult patients receiving second doses experience severe local reactions. A longer period of observation and further field trials are necessary before the usefulness of booster doses is firmly established.

SIDE-EFFECTS AND ADVERSE REACTIONS TO VACCINATION

Children who receive the vaccine may experience pain, erythema, and induration at the site of injection, and a small number may have mild fever. Most have little or no reaction. However, severe systemic reactions consisting of prolonged high fever, shaking chills, marked warmth, swelling, induration, and tenderness at the vaccination site have been reported to occur in adult patients and on rare occasions, in children. No fatality has been attributed to vaccination.

There have been several case reports of vaccinated children and adult patients vaccinated because they were at risk for pneumococcal infection who experienced bacteremia with strains included in the vaccine. Two cases have occurred in children with nephrotic syndromes. In one case, a 4-year-old boy with nephrotic syndrome on prednisone treatment developed type 4 pneumococcal sepsis. He did not demonstrate an antibody response to the type 4 antigen in the vaccine although he had responded to 7 of 11 vaccine types assayed. In the other case, type 19A sepsis developed in a 4-year-old girl who was not on immunosuppressive therapy; her vaccine contained type 19F antigen, which is related and probably cross-protective. A recent case of 6A sepsis occurred in a 25-year-old woman with Hodgkin's disease after splenectomy, completion of therapy, and vaccination (in that order). Serologic analysis demonstrated no response to the vaccine type 6A antigen.

Clearly, pneumococcal infections caused by nonvaccine strains will continue to occur and cannot be prevented.

The practical meaning of these observations is that children who receive pneumococcal polysaccharide vaccine remain susceptible to bacteremia and therefore must *also* receive ongoing antibiotic prophylaxis and prompt, vigorous treatment for any infectious episode. Physicians should also remember that asplenic and immunocompromised patients may experience serious infections with nonpneumococcal organisms, especially *Hemophilus influenzae.* Thus, administration of pneumococcal vaccine should not give one a false sense of security.

REFERENCES

Ahonkhai VI, Landesman SH, Fikrig SM et al: Failure of pneumococcal vaccine in children with sickle cell disease. N Engl J Med 301:26– 27, 1979

Broome CV, Facklam RR, Allen JR et al: Epidemiology of pneumococcal serotypes in the United States, 1978– 1979. J Infect Dis 141:119– 123, 1980

Broome CV, Facklam RR, Fraser DW: Pneumococcal disease after pneumococcal vaccination: An alternative method to estimate the efficacy of pneumococcal vaccine. N Engl J Med 303:549– 552, 1980

Center for Disease Control: Pneumococcal polysaccharide vaccine. Morb Mort Week Rep 27:25– 31, 1978

Cowan MJ, Ammann AJ, Wara DW et al: Pneumococcal polysaccharide immunization in infants and children. Pediatrics 62:721– 726, 1978

Gray BN, Converse GM III, Dillon HC Jr: Serotypes of *Streptococcus pneumoniae* causing disease. J Infect Dis 140:979– 983, 1979

Guckian JC, Christensen GD, Fine DP: The role of opsonins in recovery from experimental pneumococcal pneumonia. J Infect Dis 142:175– 190, 1980

Jacobs MR, Koornhof HJ, Robins-Browne RM et al: Emergence of multiply resistant pneumococci. New Engl J Med 299:735– 740, 1978

Klein JO, Mortimer EA: Use of pneumococcal vaccine in children. Pediatrics 61:321– 322, 1978

Lauer BA, Reller LB: Serotypes and penicillin susceptibility of pneumococci isolated from blood. J Clin Microbiol 11:242– 244, 1980

Makela PW, Herra E, Sibakov M et al: Pneumococcal vaccine and otitis media. Lancet i:547– 551, 1980

Moore DH, Shackelford PG, Robson AM et al: Recurrent pneumococcal sepsis and defective opsonization after pneumococcal capsular polysaccharide vaccine in a child with nephrotic syndrome. J Pediatr 96:882– 886, 1980

Mufson MA, Kruss DM, Wasil RE et al: Capsular types and outcome of bacteremic pneumococcal disease in the antibiotic era. Arch Intern Med 134:505– 510, 1974

Primack WA, Rosel M, Thirumoorthi MC: Failure of pneumococcal vaccine to prevent *Streptococcus pneumoniae* sepsis in nephrotic children. Lancet ii:1192, 1979

Saah AJ, Mallonnee JP, Tarpay M et al: Relative resistance to penicillin in the pneumococcus. JAMA 243:1824– 1827, 1980

Siegel JD, Poziviak CS, Michaels RH: Serotypically defined pneumococcal infections in children. J Pediatr 93:249– 250, 1978

Uhl G, Farber J, Moench T: Febrile reactions to pneumococcal vaccine. Lancet ii:1318, 1978

21

Meningococcal Infections

James F. Jones

DISEASE

Neisseria meningitidis, a gram-negative diplococcus, is responsible for a variety of clinical syndromes; the most serious are meningitis and meningococcemia. Although bacteremia always accompanies meningitis, the converse is not true; meningococcemia accompanied by purpura and shock may be fulminating and unassociated with meningeal seeding. In the United States, these illnesses occur primarily in young children and in military recruits.

Other meningococcal clinical syndromes include conjunctivitis, bacteremia associated with mild illness, arthritis, pleuritis, pneumonia, pericarditis, urethritis, epididymitis, and tracheitis.

The incidence of each type of clinical disease is low; the overall incidence of meningococcal infection in the United States is one per 100,000 population. In the "meningitis belt" of Africa, however, attack rates may be as high as one per 1000 population. The attack rate is much lower than the rates of infection or carrier state; only 10% of those who are infected actually manifest clinical illness.

Meningococci are divisible into discrete serotypes including A, B, C, D, X, Y, Z, W-135, and 29E. In the United States in the past, most disease was caused by serogroups A, B, C, and Y. Meningitis and meningococcemia occur in both sporadic and epidemic forms; groups C and B have been responsible for most sporadic disease in the United States, and group A has been described in a skid-row epidemic in Seattle, Washington.

In a recent typical year (1975), the Center for Disease Control (CDC) recorded 1478 cases of which 333 (22.5%) occurred in infants and 358 (24.2%) in children 1 to 4 years of age. Currently, most cases in the United States are sporadic and are caused by sulfa-sensitive serogroup B organisms. Group C accounts for a third of cases but the highly age-specific group C disease occurs in infancy.

IMMUNIZING ANTIGEN

The outer layer of *N. meningitidis* contains a variety of antigenic substances. Proteins, lipopolysaccharides, and polysaccharides trigger an immune response in infected persons. The polysaccharides of serogroups A, B, and C induce specific antibodies that have been associated with specific immunity. Even though cross-reacting antibodies may be evoked, protection against infection has been correlated with bactericidal antibodies against group-specific polysaccharides. Liquid cultures of group-specific organisms are treated with detergent in order to separate capsular, polysaccharide molecules from nucleic acids and protein. The polysaccharides of groups A and C that are identified as polymers of N-acetyl-O-acetylmannosamine phosphate and N-acetyl-O-acetylneuraminic acid, respectively, are supplied as freeze-dried powder that is reconstituted with isotonic sodium chloride and preserved with 1 : 10,000 thiomersol.

Polysaccharides from groups B, Y, W135, and 29E have also been isolated. Purified group B polysaccharide, primarily N-acetyl-neuraminic acid, has not proved to be immunogenic in humans, whereas preparations of the others do evoke antibody production.

Protein components from group B organisms are effective as immunogens. This is not surprising, because all three types of antigens (protein, lipopolysaccharide, and polysaccharide) stimulate immune responses in infected persons. However, in all vaccine studies, the polysaccharide components have been used.

Vaccines currently available include monovalent group A, monovalent group C, and combined groups A and C.

RATIONALE FOR IMMUNIZATION

Although the incidence of infection with meningococcus is low compared with infection with other bacteria, the outcome can be devastating. In 1978, the incidence of bacterial meningitis caused by *N. meningitidis* was 0.72 per 100,000, and the incidence for *Haemophilus influenzae* was 1.25 per 100,000; the case-to-fatality ratio, however, was 13.5% versus 7.1% respectively. There have also been epidemics of *N. meningitidis* infection. The spread of the organism is rapid, with high disease rates in restricted population groups such as military training camps. There have been massive epidemics recently in Finland and South America.

If a safe, effective vaccine were available, it could be deployed both in specific high-risk population groups and across entire populations if epidemic risk were predictable.

IMMUNITY

Resolution of meningococcal infection is associated with production of specific antibodies directed against the three outer membrane components as described above. Antibody serves as an opsonin with increased efficiency of phagocytosis and is also bactericidal for the organism. Patients who lack the eighth component of complement have chronic or recurrent infections with *N. meningitidis,* suggesting a role for the terminal attack sequence in the complement cascade in extraphagocyte killing.

Natural protection against disease also occurs. Nasopharyngeal carriage of any of the typeable or nontypeable groups results in the development of antibodies that cross-react with all types of meningococcus. Other bacteria, such as *Escherichieae coli* and *H. influenzae,* with polysaccharide capsular or other cell wall antigens that are similar to those of *N. meningitidis,* also produce cross-reacting antibodies that are protective. Many infants carry *Neisseria lactamica,* an avirulent neisseria species that crossreacts with the major antigens of *N. meningitidis* and *H. influenzae* type B.

The acquisition of antibodies against groups A and C occurs at different times in childhood. Presumed protective levels (1 to 2 μg/ml) of anti-A are reached in 90% of children by 7 months of age, whereas the same degree of antibody rates against group C organisms is not reached until 6 to 8 years of age. These data suggest that contact with group A meningococci and with other organisms bearing cross-reactive antigens occurs early in life. Contact with group C meningococci is less likely in infancy. Group A and C meningococci usually do not establish carrier states in children unless there is close contact with military personnel, in whom group C organisms are more prevalent.

SCHEDULING OF IMMUNIZATION

Routine immunization with meningococcal vaccines is not recommended.

Epidemics of group A or C disease can be controlled by planned massive immunization programs. Group A vaccine aided in aborting an epidemic in Brazil in persons more than 1 year old. Similarly, group C vaccine successfully prevented an epidemic in Finland in infants and children 3 months to 5 years of age. Group A vaccine has been used in epidemic control in the continental United States and in Alaska.

Group C vaccine has been routinely administered to all military recruits since 1971.

Anyone planning to visit areas of epidemic meningococcal disease of types A or C can be given vaccine of the appropriate type prior to leaving.

Some authorities recommend giving the appropriate monovalent vaccine to family contacts of anyone infected with group A or C strains. Half of secondary cases occur more than 5 days after the contact case. Chemoprophylaxis (either rifampin or sulfa, depending on the sensitivity pattern) should always be administered to household contacts.

The dose and route of vaccination are as specified by the manufacturer.

SPECIAL CIRCUMSTANCES FOR USE OF VACCINE

Single group A and C vaccinations effectively immunize adult patients. Protective levels in children less than 5 years old may be attained if they are immunized with group A vaccine before 3 months of age and boosters are given at 18 and 24 months of age, and again between ages 4 to 6 years. Since there is little disease of this type in the United States, this schedule is not currently recommended.

The group C vaccine is not effective in immunizing children under 2 years of age and may actually induce tolerance; it is therefore not recommended for routine use.

There is no currently available vaccine against group B, the other major neurologic pathogen in children. Because infections from other group-specific meningococci are rare, specific vaccine development and use is not warranted at this time.

SIDE-EFFECTS

Side-effects from meningococcal vaccines are minimal. If administered intradermally, A and C vaccines cause erythema, swelling, and tenderness at the injection site that usually disappear within 24 hours. Subcutaneous administration does not produce any local reactions. Fever is rare; less than 2% of 1.2 million persons receiving group A vaccine had a temperature of greater than 38.5°C (101.2°F). It has been suggested that endotoxin contamination of some vaccines may have rendered them pyrogenic.

ADVERSE REACTIONS

One theoretic problem in the development of polysaccharide vaccines is the ability of polysaccharide antigens to induce tolerance (immune paralysis). Usually, large amounts of antigen must be given repetitively in order to produce tolerance. During the development of group A vaccines, several lots also contained small amounts of group C antigen. This material was administered to volunteers who received group C vaccine two weeks later. Surprisingly, no antibody response to group C antigen was detected six weeks after immunization. This phenomenon suggests the induction of tolerance and underscores the care that must be exercised in the development and use of polysaccharide vaccines.

Theoretically, uneven use of group-specific vaccines could result in the emergence of disease caused by other groups. This phenomenon has not been observed thus far in the use of meningococcal vaccine.

REFERENCES

Artenstein MS, Gold R, Zimmerly JG et al: Prevention of meningococcal disease by group C polysaccharide vaccine. N Engl J Med 282:417, 1970

Baltimore RS, Hammerschlag M: Meningococcal bacteremia: Clinical and serological studies of infants with mild disease. Am J Dis Child 131:1001, 1977

Brandt BL, Artenstein MD: Duration of antibody responses after vaccination with group C *Neisseria meningitidis* polysaccharide. J Infect Dis 131:569, 1975

Center for Disease Control: Bacterial meningitis and meningococcemia. Morb Mort Week Rep 28:277, 1979

Editorial: Who should be given meningococcal vaccine? Lancet 2:1185, 1978

Evans-Jones LG, Whittle HC, Onyewotu II et al: Comparative study of group A and group C meningococcal infection. Arch Dis Child 52:320, 1977

Geldman HA: Some recollections of the meningoccal diseases. JAMA 220:1107, 1972

Glode MP, Robbins JB, Liu T-Y et al: Cross-antigenicity and immunogenicity between capsular polysaccharides of group C *Neisseria meningitidis* and of *Escherichia coli* K92. J Infect Dis 135:94, 1977

Gold R: Polysaccharide meningoccal vaccines—current status. Hosp Pract 14:41–48, 1979

Gold R, Goldschneider I, Lepow ML et al: Carriage of *Neisseria meningitidis* and *Neisseria lactamica* in infants and children. J Infect Dis 137:112, 1978

Gold R, Lepow ML, Goldschneider I et al: Kinetics of antibody production to group A and group C meningococcal polysaccharide vaccines administered during the first six years of life: Prospects for routine administration of infants and children. J Infect Dis 140:690, 1979

Greenwood BM, Hassan-King M, Whittle HC: Prevention of secondary cases of meningococcal disease in household contacts by vaccination. Br Med J 1:1317, 1978

Greenwood BM, Wali SS: Control of meningococcal infection in the African meningitis belt by selective vaccination. Lancet 1:729, 1980

Lepow ML, Goldschneider I, Gold R et al: Persistance of antibody following immunization of children with groups A and C meningococcal polysaccharide vaccines. Pediatrics 60:673, 1977

Makela PH, Kayhty H, Weckstrom P et al: Effect of group A meningococcal vaccine in army recruits in Finland. Lancet 2:883, 1975

Marks MI, Frasch CE, Shapera RM: Meningococcal colonization and infection in children and their household contacts. Am J Epidemiol 109:563, 1979

Monto AS, Brandt BL, Artenstein MS: Response of children to *Neisseria meningitidis* polysaccharide vaccines. J Infect Dis 127:394, 1973

Wilkins J, Wehrle PF: Further characterization of responses of infants and children to meningococcal A polysaccharide vaccine. J Pediatr 94:828, 1979

Zollinger WD, Mandrell RE, Altieri P et al: Safety and immunogenicity of a *Neisseria meningitidis* type 2 protein vaccine in animals and humans. J Infect Dis 137:728, 1978

22

Less Frequently Used Vaccines

Vincent A. Fulginiti

Certain vaccines are not included in routine recommended immunizations for infants and children. In general, these vaccines are given to specific groups for specific reasons and the clinician is urged to consult up-to-date sources at the time the need for such vaccines appears to be indicated. For example, as this chapter was being prepared, typhus vaccine was included because it was then available. Later in the course of this chapter's preparation, the vaccine was removed from the market, and thus its description is deleted here. This and similar episodes point to the need for constantly updating the information about the vaccines included in this chapter.

CHOLERA VACCINE

In recent years, cholera has been due to the El Tor biotype, and has been epidemic throughout much of Asia, the Middle East, and Africa, and in certain parts of Europe. During the past two years, isolated cases have been reported in the United States. Cholera is acquired primarily by ingestion of *Vibrio cholera* in contaminated water or food, particularly seafood. Ordinary travel abroad, even to endemic areas, is usually not associated with a significant risk of contracting this disease.

Cholera vaccine currently available to physicians in the United States is prepared by an activation of two classic strains grown *in vitro*. The vaccine is inactivated chemically, usually with phenol, and is intended for intradermal, subcutaneous, or intramuscular administration.

Indications for use of cholera vaccine are limited to the following circumstances: (1) prolonged residence in endemic areas; (2) sustained

TABLE 22-1. Cholera Vaccine: Age-Determined Route and Dose

Age	Dose	Route
5 yr and over	0.2 ml	Intradermal*
6 mo– 4 yr	0.2 ml	Subcutaneous or intramuscular
5– 10 yr	0.3 ml	Subcutaneous or intramuscular
over 10 yr	0.5 ml	Subcutaneous or intramuscular

* Use of intradermal vaccine is to avoid significant reactions. If a higher level of protection is desirable, the subcutaneous or intramuscular route according to the table should be employed.

travel through endemic areas where contact with contaminated water or food is likely; and (3) extensive exposure to the vibrio such as that experienced by laboratory workers.

Occasionally, specific occupations may necessitate cholera immunization as a condition of employment. Unfortunately, some countries require that travelers have proof of cholera immunization even though no clear-cut recommendation exists for such persons. Thus, some physicians may be confronted with a contradiction, in that they will be asked to administer a vaccine for which the experts indicate no need.

Infants under 6 months of age should not receive cholera vaccine, nor should it be given to anyone who has had a serious reaction to a previous dose. Under these circumstances, the physician may have to provide the traveler with documentation of a medical contraindication to vaccination. Because it is uncertain whether pregnancy is adversely affected by cholera vaccine, the physician is urged to be cautious in vaccinating pregnant women and such action should be taken only in high-risk situations.

A complete primary series of cholera vaccine is only indicated for persons in these risk categories. If the only indication for cholera vaccination is that it is required by the country to which the patient is traveling, a single dose will suffice.

The usual regimen involves a primary series of two doses or a booster dose within six months if the primary series has been received within that interval. The route and dose are age-determined as shown in Table 22-1.

Booster doses are 0.2 ml for the intradermal route and the same doses by age as used for the subcutaneous or intramuscular route in the table above. The two doses should be separated by one to four weeks or longer. Booster doses may be given every six months if necessary but may be discontinued if the occurrence of cholera is episodic. The resumption of booster doses should continue prior to the next cholera season.

I have had, and seen others have, severe reactions to cholera vaccine. Although such reactions are not the norm, many patients will experience one to two days of local pain, redness, and induration at the injection site. Fever, generalized achiness, and malaise during the same period are not uncommon. In severe reactions, all of these symptoms are exaggerated and may be prolonged for a few days. In some instances, bed rest may be necessary.

PLAGUE VACCINE

Plague is currently endemic in the western United States, particularly in the Four Corners area of Utah, Colorado, New Mexico, and Arizona, and in California. In many other parts of the world, plague is endemic because of infection in rodents and their accompanying ectoparasites. Endemic and epidemic plague is currently encountered in Africa, Asia, and in some parts of South America.

Plague vaccine is prepared from artificially grown *Yersinia pestis*, inactivated with formaldehyde and preserved with phenol. The vaccine is injected intramuscularly.

Immunization against plague is recommended for the following: (1) laboratory and other workers who come in contact with plague organisms, particularly if the organisms are resistant to antimicrobial agents (some experts feel that plague vaccine should be administered only to persons working with resistant organisms); (2) persons engaged in experiments involving aerosols of *Yersinia pestis;* (3) persons working in areas of disaster or in other field operations where plague is endemic and exposure cannot be controlled; (4) less definitely, anyone living or working in endemic or epidemic areas who may have contact with infected ectoparasites; and (5) anyone whose occupation results in regular contact with wild rodents, rabbits, or other lagomorphs in areas where plague is prevalent.

In children less than 10 years old, three doses of vaccine are administered and booster doses given at approximately 6-month intervals to a total of 5 doses. A similar schedule is followed in adult patients and in children more than 10 years old as shown in Table 22-2.

With a regimen of five doses, almost all recipients will have protective levels of antibody (titers of 1 : 128 or higher). *Booster doses* to maintain immunity may be given at one to two year intervals.

The exact effectiveness of plague vaccine is indeterminate. Its long use simply suggests that the incidence and severity of plague in immunized persons is reduced.

Many experience tenderness, redness, and induration at the injection site. With subsequent doses, vague general systemic symptoms and

TABLE 22-2. Plague Vaccine: Schedule of Doses

Age	First Two Doses	Third Dose and All Booster Doses
Older than 10 yr	0.5 ml	0.2 ml
5– 10 yr	0.3 ml	0.12 ml
1– 4 yr	0.2 ml	0.08 ml
Less than 1 yr	0.1 ml	0.04 ml

fever may occur and may increase in severity. Serious complications have not been recorded.

TYPHUS VACCINE

Typhus has not been experienced in the United States since 1950, and epidemic typhus, not since 1922. World-wide, typhus is decreasing in incidence, probably because of improved living conditions and the extensive use of insecticides to control lice. Recently, typhus vaccine was withdrawn from production and is no longer available in the United States.

ANTHRAX VACCINE

The agent of anthrax, *Bacillus anthracis,* is endemic in certain parts of the world. Exposure in this country is primarily an occupational hazard of workers who process hides, hair, bone, wool, and animal product fertilizer; of veterinarians; and of agricultural workers who handle infected animals. Anthrax is infrequent and sporadic; rare, nonoccupational cases have occurred in home craftsmen working with contaminated yarn. In 1978, six cases of human cutaneous anthrax were reported, four in industrial settings and two in agricultural ones.

The vaccine is a cell-free, alum-precipitated antigen prepared from sterile culture filtrates in which the Rl-NP mutant of the Volum strain of *B. anthracis* is grown. This mutant is nonproteolytic and unencapsulated.

Vaccination is reserved for those at high risk of exposure. An antibody response may be expected in anyone older than 6 months of age. Three subcutaneous doses of 0.5 ml are given at two to three week intervals, with an annual 0.5-ml booster.

Reactions include local edema, induration, warmth, tenderness, and pruritis, with occasional systemic malaise. Immunization of people in contact with cases is unnecessary, and immunization of children would almost never be indicated.

TULAREMIA VACCINE

Infection with *Francisella tularensis* causes tularemia. The organism is found in infected wild and domestic animals and in the ticks, flies, and other insects that bite them. Inoculation occurs through skin or conjunctiva directly or by the bites of infected insects. It may also occur through ingestion of contaminated water or of an infected and inadequately cooked animal, or through inhalation. Infection occurs readily among laboratory personnel working with the organism.

F. tularensis is a facultative intracellular parasite; in animals, immunity depends largely on cellular rather than humoral mechanisms. Even documented infection with virulent organisms does not prevent reinfection.

Immunization is only recommended for those at high risk of infection, such as laboratory workers; children almost never need tularemia immunization. The vaccine consists of live attenuated bacteria produced from a colony-type variant of *F. tularensis*. Immunization does not prevent entirely, but does reduce substantially, the incidence of typhoidal tularemia. The occurrence of ulceroglandular tularemia remains the same but the severity of this disease is decreased.

One drop of vaccine is administered by means of multiple punctures. Local inflammation occurs and healing with scarring and occasional enlargement of regional lymph nodes ensues, but no systemic reaction is encountered. Inoculation of contacts of cases is unnecessary.

MIXED BACTERIAL VACCINES

From time to time, reports appear touting the effectiveness of spontaneously made "mixed bacterial vaccines" for patients with allergic diseases, principally asthma. Proponents of this approach cite "bacterial allergy" as a cause for exacerbation of the allergic disease and claim vaccine administration is of benefit in reducing sensitivity to bacterial antigens.

There is no substantive proof of either the theory of bacterial allergy or of the effectiveness of such vaccines. I do not recommend their use.

REFERENCES

Bartelloni PJ, Marshall JD Jr, Cavanaugh DC: Clinical and serologic responses to plague vaccine, USP. Milit Med 138:720–722, 1973

Barus D, Burrows W (eds): Cholera. Philadelphia, WB Saunders, 1974

Brachman PS, Gold H, Plotkin SA et al: Field evaluation of human anthrax vaccine. Am J Publ Health 52:632–645, 1962

Burke DS: Immunization against tularemia. J Infect Dis 136:55–60, 1977

Center for Disease Control: Cholera vaccine. Morb Mort Week Rep 27:173, 1978

Center for Disease Control: Plague vaccine. Morb Mort Week Rep 27:255, 1978

Phillippines Cholera Committee: A controlled field trial on the effectiveness of the intradermal and subcutaneous administration of cholera vaccine in the Phillipines. Bull WHO 49:389–394, 1973

Sommer A, Khan M, Mosley WH: Efficacy of vaccination of family contacts of cholera cases. Lancet 1:1230–1232, 1973

23
Immune Globulin (IG)

Vincent A. Fulginiti

Immune globulin (IG) has been described in detail in Chapter 2. This pharmaceutical has been termed "immune serum globulin," "poliomyelitis immune globulin," "normal serum immune globulin," and so forth. Its official designation is immune globulin (IG). It is a ±16.5% concentrated solution of gamma-phoretic globulins prepared from pooled human plasma obtained from a large number of donors. It contains principally IgG (95%+) and only trace amounts of IgA, IgM, and other human serum proteins.

The basic principle for the use of IG lies in its heterogeneous content of antibody. Obtained from 1000 or more adult donors, its antibody content reflects their collective antigenic experience. Predictably, it will contain large quantities of measles antibody, hepatitis A antibody, and an assortment of other antibodies. Since 1972, hepatitis-B-antigen-positive donors have been eliminated. Lots of IG since that time have contained at least some hepatitis B antibody as a result of this exclusion; titers have not varied since 1977.

It will be necessary, in the future, to continuously assay the antibody content of IG preparations. As the epidemiology of various diseases changes, as detailed in the specific disease sections, the antibody content in donated plasma will vary. Thus, it will become necessary to be certain that enough measles or other specific antibodies are present to ensure the desired prophylactic effect. The fact that all preparations contain a variety of antibacterial, antitoxic, and some antiviral antibodies, makes an IG useful as replacement therapy for those who lack their own antibody, such as patients with congenital hypogamma-globulinemia. The predictable amount of specific antibodies makes IG useful in specific disease prophylaxis such as measles-neutralizing antibody in prevention of measles.

PHARMACOLOGY OF IMMUNE GLOBULIN

Immune globulin delivers IgG to the recipient. Efficient serum levels are achieved within two days following intramuscular injection. From peak levels, the IgG decays with a half-life in the range of 22 to 28 days. For most antibodies, the serum level is reduced below effective amounts within two to three half lives. For this reason, one can effectively immunize a susceptible person who received IG with live virus vaccine three months later.

The IgG in IG is distributed in approximately 2.2 times the plasma volume, reaching the interstitial fluid. It does not enter the cerebrospinal fluid (CSF) unless there is a "protein leak" such as occurs in inflammatory disease of the meninges. Immune globulin is relatively inert in relation to host responsiveness. At its ±16.5% concentration, it is a local irritant. Administration is often accompanied by local pain and tenderness even when given properly in a large muscle mass. Volumes larger than 5 ml are poorly tolerated and this is the maximum that should be given at any one site. In infants and young children, one may wish to limit this volume further to 2 to 3 ml maximum at any one site.

Intramuscular administration is the only acceptable route. This is a highly viscous solution and should be administered with a large bore needle. A large muscle mass should be selected. In many younger patients the vastus lateralis is acceptable and injection in the anterolateral thigh is preferred. In older individuals, the deltoid muscle mass may be large enough. In many cases, it will be necessary to administer gamma-globulin into the buttocks. If the gluteal region is selected, great care must be taken to ensure that there is no injury to the sciatic nerve or blood vessels (see Chapter 3).

Intradermal administration usually produces a nonspecific wheal and flare reaction that is of no specific immunologic significance or value to the patient; *this route is not indicated for any purpose.* Subcutaneous administration may result in severe irritation secondary to the concentration of the solution. Immune globulin should never be administered by this route deliberately. Care should be taken to prevent inadvertent leakage of IG from the site of intramuscular injection. The usual method is to deflect the skin and subcutaneous tissues laterally over the anticipated muscle injection site; following the injection, the skin is allowed to spring back to its original position, disconnecting the injection tract at the subcutaneous muscle interface (the Z method; see Chapter 3).

The intravenous route is contraindicated for IG. No preparation currently available commercially in the United States should be given intravenously. Such preparations are highly anticomplementary; IgG molecules aggregate into dimers and polymers and behave as if antigen were linking them. They fix complement and can result in anaphylaxis if injected intravenously. Polymerization occurs upon storage of this concentrated solution.

Attempts have been made to render gammaglobulin preparations safe for intravenous use. In the past, enzyme digestion and other methods have been employed in an attempt to facilitate intravenous administration. A new technique, mild reduction and alkylation, preserves the Fc' region of IgG, which is altered in the enzyme-treated preparations. This new intravenous preparation has a half-life of 20 days and retains more than 80% of antibody activity. Importantly, it can be administered intravenously with minimal reaction. In one study, a third of recipients experienced mild transient fever, nausea, flushing, and muscle cramping during infusion. None experienced persistent or severe reactions. This product is currently experimental and is not commercially available in the United States.

Other intravenous preparations are also in trials or clinical use in various parts of the world. Acid treatment and sulphonation have been used in an attempt to manufacture these intravenous gammaglobulins.

ADVERSE REACTIONS TO IMMUNE GLOBULIN

Apart from local irritation at the intramuscular site of injection, most people experience few side-effects to IG. Anaphylactic reactions, which are rare, may be the result of inadvertent intravenous administration. Alternatively, anaphylaxis may be related to intramuscular administration. In a 10 year observation period in England, 85 reactions were noted among 40,000 injections; 33 (19%) of 175 recipients reacted. This experience has not been duplicated on a smaller scale among any group of patients receiving IG.

Chills, nausea, a feeling of apprehension, and flushing within a period of up to 30 minutes after receiving IG are not uncommon. Occasionally, patients will also vomit and become cyanotic. Cardiovascular collapse and unconsciousness can occur in severe reactions. In some instances, these reactions are transient and mild; in others, they are severe and progressive. It is impossible to determine the course an individual patient will follow. Hence, therapy for anaphylaxis is recommended to include immediate epinephrine administration and antihistaminic treatment (see Chapter 2).

A final possible cause of hypersensitivity reactions is mercury sensitivity. It has been known for some time that mercury accumulates in recipients of IG over long intervals. In one case reported, acrodynia developed because the patient had become sensitive to mercury after prolonged exposure to the organic mercurial preservative used in IG. Symptoms included a pink rash on the palms and soles, flushed cheeks, photophobia, irritability, a fine tremor, and altered sensation in the fingertips.

Despite the potential for adverse immunologic reactions to IG, few have been noted. Immune globulin contains all subclasses of IgG and all Gm genetic types (see Chapter 2). Clinical reactions are rare. Since IG contains trace amounts of IgA, anti-IgA antibodies may develop in a recipient who is selectively deficient for IgA. I treated one patient who experienced febrile reactions with chills and other features of anaphylaxis after receiving IG. These reactions were believed to be related to anti-IgA antibodies detected in her serum. Although generally hypogammaglobulinemic, she completely lacked any detectable level of serum IgA. Once sensitized by IG, such a patient is also at risk from receipt of blood containing IgA; if sensitized by a previous blood transfusion, patient can experience a reaction to administration of IG.

The theoretic fear that female recipients of IG might become sensitized to IgG and produce offspring with hypogammaglobulinemia has not been realized. Empiric and anecdotal observations, and one systematic attempt to detect such an event, have failed to produce a single documented instance of sensitization and disease.

SPECIFIC USES OF IMMUNE GLOBULIN

ANTIBODY-DEFICIENT INDIVIDUALS

Since Bruton first described congenital, sex-linked hypogammaglobulinemia, it has been apparent that replacement with gammaglobulin can prevent many of the infectious episodes to which patients with this disease are susceptible and can reduce the severity of those episodes that occur. In addition, other manifestations of hypogammaglobulinemia, such as persistent arthritis, also subside. Immune globulin contains a sufficient variety of specific antibodies to provide the antibody-deficient patient with passive protection by repetitive administration.

Since IG only provides systemic IgG, no relief from mucosal infections is anticipated or realized. Those receiving IG may still have otitis media, sinobronchial infections, and recurrent or persistent pneumonia.

It should be noted that IG can be used whenever there is an antibody deficiency, whether congenital or acquired. Thus, those with diminished antibody-synthesizing capacity from other congenital and acquired causes should also be considered candidates for IG administration. It is beyond the scope of this text to detail such conditions. The reader is referred to the immunologic references at the end of this chapter.

In the United States, IG can be obtained through the American Red Cross. It is also commercially available but it is very expensive, a milliliter costing between $1 and $5 in 1980. The dosage of IG to be used in antibody deficiencies varies. The most common working guideline is to use an initial dose of approximately 230 mg (1.4 ml) of IG/kg of body weight. Following the initial loading dose, half that amount or 115 mg/kg (0.7 ml) is administered monthly. The effectiveness of such therapy will vary considerably. The goal is to eliminate serious infectious diseases such as pneumococcal bacteremia and meningitis, which have usually occurred prior to IG administration. Some patients will need larger amounts of IG than the standard guidelines suggest. Most commonly, the increased dose is accommodated by increasing the frequency of administration and keeping each dose at the 0.7 ml/kg level. The maximum dose should not exceed 20 to 30 ml per administration. It is seldom necessary to administer IG more often than every three weeks. However, on rare occasions, it may be necessary to resort to a 10-day interval.

The Medical Research Council in England demonstrated that 50 mg/kg/week of IG administered to patients with antibody deficiencies resulted in significantly fewer infections than occurred in those who received the standard dose of 25 mg/kg/week. The latter dose had been selected, in part, because of the convenient volume in which it was delivered. Larger volumes were uncomfortable to administer and therefore never became part of standard practice. It is equally interesting that antibody-deficient patients receiving intravenous preparations of gammaglobulin appear to do better when the dose is 150 mg/kg/month. Unfortunately, these dosage levels, which appear to have significant clinical benefit, cannot be achieved easily with intramuscular administration. As a result, the lower doses continue to be recommended as a practical compromise between immunologic effectiveness and patient comfort and safety. Should intravenous gammaglobulin become widely available, it may be possible to administer a larger quantity of IG and to achieve a significantly better clinical effect.

Many patients with long-standing patterns of infections and IG administration can recognize when the gammaglobulin effect is "wearing off". They will report vague feelings of unease plus characteristic symptoms related to their previous patterns of infections that begin to appear as the effect of the prior dose of IG decreases below clinical effectiveness.

Only clinical criteria are used in determining IG dosage. It is clear that serum levels will not correlate with clinical effect and thus should not be used to monitor IG administration. In exceptional circumstances, the serum IgG level is used to guide therapy. For example, in one case of progressive vaccinia, I attempted to achieve normal levels of IgG in order to determine whether the viremia could be halted. In another case, specific levels of varicella antibody were measured in an attempt to halt dissemination of this virus by massive administration of various forms of passive antibody. These unusual circumstances do not pertain to the ordinary prophylaxis of patients with antibody deficiencies. In fact, administration of 115 mg of IG/kg of body weight usually increases the IgG level only slightly more than 100 mg/dl, an amount that does not correlate with the clinical effect observed. Rather, it is the specific antibody contained within that amount of IG administered that is responsible for the improved health of the patient.

MEASLES PROPHYLAXIS

Persons with serum-neutralizing antibody to measles resist infection. This long-established fact suggested to early investigators that measles antibody might be transferred to a susceptible host prior to the development of disease and result in protection. The most significant observations in this regard were made by Dr. Stokes at the University of Pennsylvania. He and his colleagues administered large doses of IG during the incubation period of measles and prevented the disease; smaller doses modified the illness. Measles antibody, given in the early stages of actual measles infection, also appeared to ameliorate the severity of the subsequent clinical disease, but this observation has been obscured with time. Others soon verified Stoke's observations, and it became relatively routine to administer IG in an effort to prevent or modify measles.

It is now evident that measles virus undergoes a replication process in the infected host which lasts for approximately 11 days prior to the appearance of clinical illness. This incubation period is extremely variable but during this phase, virus replicates in the reticuloendothelial system (RES). There appear to be two distinct phases of viremia; an early phase occurs in the first few days after exposure following replication of the virus in the respiratory tract and regional lymph nodes. This initial, low-level viremia serves to seed the entire RES, and additional replication occurs until a sufficient mass of measles virus is released into the blood coincident with the first symptoms of the disease.

Thus, the rationale for antibody administration is to provide passive neutralizing antibody during the early days of disease, preferably within the first six days after exposure, to inhibit the initial viremic spread, and thus to confine the replication of the virus to the respiratory tract and regional lymph nodes, where its effects are asymptomatic. If this is successfully accomplished, the disease may be completely aborted without evidence of systemic, permanent immunity. Alternatively, depending on the dose and timing of IG and the degree of replication and spread that the virus has already undergone, active-passive immunity without clinical disease may develop. In such cases, the patient will remain resistant to natural infection for the rest of his life.

Prior to the availability of live measles virus (LMV) vaccine, many physicians preferred to use modifying doses of IG in an attempt to provide such life-long immunity. In the modified disease, clinical symptoms were mild or negligible, complications were prevented and permanent immunity often resulted. However, some practitioners preferred to prevent measles altogether by administering large doses as soon after exposure as possible. Once LMV vaccine became available and its effectiveness was demonstrated, many, including myself, believed that modifying doses should no longer be used. The rationale behind this belief is that even in modified measles, a small degree of risk from complications remains. This small degree of risk can probably be eliminated by using the larger doses of IG and by subsequently immunizing the patient with LMV vaccine.

For prevention of measles, 0.25 ml/kg of IG should be administered intramuscularly as soon as possible after exposure. This timing is critical if there is to be maximum opportunity to prevent measles. Some argue that IG should be administered at any point during the incubation period prior to the appearance of symptoms, basing their advice upon Stoke's observation of amelioration of clinical disease with large doses. Although not advocated by myself and most recommending bodies, the modifying dose of IG is 0.1 ml/kg.

Special circumstances exist in cases of pediatric leukemia and other malignancies as well as in children who are immunodeficient (particularly in T cells) or who are receiving immunosuppressive therapy. Severe, even fatal, disease has been observed in such children with measles virus infection. Similarly, LMV administration in such children has caused severe infection and even death. As a result, a susceptible child in one of these categories should receive immunoprophylaxis in the form of IG. Some experts argue for administration only upon known exposure. However, others point out that not all exposures are detectable and that if measles is prevalent, the child should receive monthly injections of IG during the interval of measles activity. Still others argue for continuous monthly injections of IG during the period of immunodeficiency. (Obviously, children with continuous immunodeficiencies who are being treated with IG do not need specific measles prophylaxis because their ordinary dosage will protect them.) Children in the categories described should receive larger doses of IG, 0.5 to 1.0 ml/kg of body weight. The upper limit of IG in such cases is 15 to 20 ml as a total dose, divided into 5-ml injections. Children who have significant thrombocytopenia or other coagulopathy may be unable to receive large doses of intramuscular IG. If possible, one of the experimental intravenous preparations should be used. If such preparations become commercially available, they will be extremely useful in the isolated instances of patients needing IG who also have bleeding disorders.

HEPATITIS PROPHYLAXIS

Immune globulin is useful in both hepatitis A and hepatitis B prophylaxis. The rationale here is that either agent can be neutralized following exposure if an appropriate dose of an antibody preparation containing sufficient amounts of specific antibody is administered. Some experts maintain that as many as 95% of patients can be protected against hepatitis A if IG is given up to 6 days before the appearance of jaundice. The effectiveness in cases of hepatitis B is more controversial and recommendations vary. This section will explore IG use in both types of hepatitis. There is no evidence for IG effectiveness in non-A, non-B hepatitis (NANB, hepatitis C).

Hepatitis A

The incubation period of hepatitis A virus infection ranges from 14 to 45 days with an average of about 25 to 30 days to the onset of clinical disease, generally the appearance of jaundice. Thus, there is a long interval during which the virus is in sufficiently susceptible form and access to permit antibody prophylaxis. All lots of IG since 1977 appear capable of preventing overt hepatitis A infection if administered any time during the incubation period prior to 6 days before the appearance of jaundice. Immune globulin appears to be ineffective if given 2 weeks or more after exposure and its use in this circumstance is not indicated. With clear-cut and known exposure, this determination may be relatively straightforward. When there have been multiple exposures or when the specific source is unknown, most experts feel it is wise to administer IG regardless of the interval in the hope that it will be within the effective period.

The dose of IG is in part dependent on the degree of exposure. There has been much confusion and disagreement about the precise dose and the definition of risk. The doses in this chapter are, in general, those conjointly agreed upon by the American Academy of Pediatrics and the CDC with some variation, which is indicated. Some expert opinions will differ for both the indications and the actual dosage.

Isolated contacts of brief duration ordinarily do not indicate any prophylaxis. For example, schoolmates attending ordinary elementary through college level classes need not receive IG if one of their classmates develops hepatitis A. Similarly, *in most daycare and nursery school situations*, single exposures need not result in massive application of IG prophylaxis. However, in epidemic situations which appear to be classroom centered, the use of IG should be considered. I have found that the best rule is to examine the specific situation to determine if household-type contact has occurred. By that it is meant opportunity for fecal-oral contamination or spread, and communal use of toilet facilities, dishes, towels, and other such fomites that might facilitate transmission. In daycare centers, the presence of children in diapers constitutes such exposure. The dose to be used in such circumstances is 0.02 ml/kg administered once.

In custodial or residential institutions, the incidence of hepatitis A is often extremely high and the risk of contracting the disease almost universal. In such circumstances, IG prophylaxis for both children and attendants appears warranted; a high-degree-exposure dose of 0.06 to 0.12 ml/kg should be given every three months (the CDC recommends 0.02 ml/kg). In an acute-care hospital, IG should not be used routinely for either patients or hospital personnel. One may wish to use the higher dose listed above for individual patients at high risk of contracting the disease and suffering its complications. An individual decision should be made in every instance.

If contaminated food, milk, or other liquids results in a common source epidemic, IG is generally ineffective except among household contacts of those who have contracted the disease.

Newborn infants whose mothers have hepatitis A virus infection during pregnancy should not be given IG unless the mother is jaundiced at the time of delivery. A dose of 0.02 ml/kg of body weight may be administered to the newborn infant; the effectiveness of this procedure is uncertain.

Short-term travel, even to areas of high endemnicity, ordinarily does not necessitate IG prophylaxis. However, if the occupation, the length of time, or the degree of exposure anticipated is such that risk of exposure to hepatitis A is high, the traveler should receive 0.02 ml/kg of IG if exposure will be for less than three months and 0.06 ml/kg if a longer stay is anticipated. This latter dose should be repeated every five months.

Animal and research workers may on rare occasions be exposed to some nonhuman primate, particularly a chimpanzee, who is infected with hepatitis A virus. Such workers should be forewarned about the risk and should obey rigid precautions concerning hand washing, particularly in handling fecal material. A 0.05 ml/kg dose of IG should be administered every five months. If facilities are available for measuring anti-hepatitis A antibody, such workers should be screened periodically; if the titer becomes positive, IG prophylaxis is no longer necessary.

In general, IG does not prevent infection with hepatitis A virus; rather, it inhibits manifestations of disease and often results in active-passive immunity. Lots of IG have varying antibody titers to hepatitis A, ranging from 1:4000 to 1:16,000. The specific antibody content may dictate whether active-passive immunity will result, although this amount of antibody is usually enough to prevent clinical disease.

On rare occasions, IG may be used in prophylaxis for a person who is accidentally inoculated with blood, serum, or other body fluids from a patient with active hepatitis A. This exposure probably warrants the larger dose, 0.06 to 0.12 ml/kg. This is a controversial use of IG and not all experts will agree to either the indication or the dosage level.

Hepatitis B

The incubation period of hepatitis B is usually 60 to 180 days with an average period of 90 days prior to the appearance of jaundice. Hepatitis B virus is transmitted most commonly by parenteral administration of blood or blood components or by inoculation of material containing hepatitis B. Although blood or blood products are usually involved, infection can also result from sexual intercourse or from ingestion of contaminated material. In rare cases, infection is caused by indirect contact with fomites or vectors. Transplacental transmission does occur in an infant born to an hepatitis-B-positive mother and jaundice may develop in the infant after birth.

High rates of infection are found among homosexuals, among those using illicit drugs, especially intravenously, among patients and personnel involved in renal dialysis, and among anyone receiving frequent blood transfusions. Both IG and specific hepatitis B immune globulin (HBIG—see Chapter 24) can be used in prophylaxis. There is considerable controversy about specific indications for the use of each of these products and for the circumstances of exposure. We will present the combined opinion of the American Academy of Pediatrics and the CDC, recognizing that others recommend deviations from these indications and dosages.

Acute minimal exposure, such as that which occurs following a scratch with a contaminated needle, splashing of infected blood into the eye or onto other mucosal surfaces, and among sexual partners, merits administration of either IG or HBIG as soon as possible after exposure. Either of these preparations should be administered within 2 days after exposure, and administration repeated in one month. The dose for either preparation is 0.05 ml/kg.

Infants whose mothers are positive for hepatitis B surface antigen during the last trimester (whether by active infection or as carriers) should receive IG prophylaxis. What is uncertain at present are the type of globulin preferred (IG versus HBIG), the dose, and the timing of administration. Conflicting studies and recommendations have clouded this area of practice.

Currently, the American Academy of Pediatrics and the CDC are recommending the following:

1. HBIG is preferred.
2. Multiple doses are preferable to a single dose.

3. Specifically:
   a. 0.5 ml/kg of HBIG should be given *as soon as possible* after birth. Many administer the globulin in the delivery room.
   b. 0.16 ml/kg of HBIG is administered at monthly intervals for a total of 5 months.

Studies of the effectiveness of this and other approaches are continuing and the final recommendation may differ. Further, some hepatitis experts vigorously espouse alternative methods. As is always the case where data are insufficient or incomplete, a variety of methods may be used. Alternatives include the following:

1. One ml of HBIG at 0, 3, and 6 months of age.
2. One ml of HBIG at 0 and 3 months of age.
3. 0.5 ml of HBIG at 0, 3, and 6 months of age.

Some advocate substituting IG for HBIG.

Those in custodial institutions and patients or personnel involved in renal dialysis should be tested for the presence of HB_sAg and those who are negative should receive IG, 0.05 to 0.07 ml/kg every four months. Testing for anti-HB_s should be repeated prior to each dose. If antibody is present, IG can be discontinued. (The CDC does not recommend routine use of IG for staff and patients. It advocates hepatitis B precautions, such as screening, segregation of carriers, and environmental hygiene. If hepatitis B is transmitted despite such measures, IG is recommended).

The reader is encouraged to keep current on IG and HBIG prophylaxis for hepatitis B. It is likely that dosages as well as recommended indications may change from time to time as more data are accumulated.

CHICKENPOX (VARICELLA) PROPHYLAXIS

For many years, it was believed that IG was of no value in the prophylaxis of varicella. The mild nature of most infections and the cost and discomfort of IG administration suggested little gain from its use. In addition, early studies reported variable success in preventing or ameliorating varicella infections in susceptible persons. It became clear that large doses of IG (up to 0.6 ml/pound of body weight) could reduce the severity of infection but not the incidence of disease. For this reason, few experts recommended IG prophylaxis under most circumstances.

Varicella-zoster infections appear to evoke a complex immunologic response in the host. Antibody alone is not the sole determinant of immunity or resistance. However, more sophisticated techniques have disclosed that a sufficient amount of antibody can result in resistance to varicella. Efforts have been made over the years to develop a specific IG containing high levels of varicella antibody. This preparation is currently known as varicella-zoster immune globulin (VZIG) and will be discussed more fully in Chapter 24.

Prophylaxis is not indicated for healthy children exposed to varicella. Adult patients and susceptible children may experience severe varicella-zoster infections. These patients should receive VZIG (see Chap. 24). For example, children with leukemia or lymphoma or those receiving immunosuppressive therapy who are susceptible to varicella may experience severe disease upon exposure; often this is a disseminated form of varicella and may be lethal.

Newborns exposed to chickenpox may also receive IG as an alternative to VZIG, although the indications here are less certain. It is known that a few newborns will develop very severe disease but for the majority in this age group, varicella is mild or even minimally apparent. Since one cannot determine the outcome for a specific infant, many prefer to administer IG in large doses (see Chapter 24 for greater detail).

RUBELLA PROPHYLAXIS

Theoretically, rubella prophylaxis by IG should be as effective as measles prophylaxis. The two viruses, although different in significant ways, do have similar replication cycles within the human host, suggesting that there is opportunity for prevention or amelioration by IG. However, specific rubella antibody in random lots of IG is varied and unpredictable. As a result, a number of studies offer contradictory evidence about IG's effectiveness in preventing rubella. In some studies, reduction in both the incidence of infection and the clinical manifestations of disease in those infected has been clearly demonstrated. In others, little or no protection against infection has been demonstrated, although clinical expression of rubella has often been inhibited. Further, IG containing a known quantity of rubella antibody (in the range of 1 : 32 to 1 : 64 neutralizing antibody titers) has had no effect in preventing rubella in experimentally inoculated volunteers or in naturally exposed patients.

These conflicting results have led some to disclaim any value for rubella prophylaxis. The only situation in which it is warranted is when a susceptible pregnant woman is exposed to natural disease during the first trimester. Others have maintained that the promising results of some studies suggest that under such circumstances, large doses of IG should be given when therapeutic abortion is deemed undesirable or is not to be considered. At the time this is written, there is no consensus between the CDC and the American Academy of Pediatrics or among various other experts. The CDC suggests that IG should not be used in rubella prophylaxis of pregnant women. The Academy has stated that it should be used with recognition that it may not be effective in some, if not most, instances.

If rubella prophylaxis is contemplated in an exposed, susceptible, pregnant woman during the first trimester, the following should be observed:

1. A serum antibody titer to rubella should be immediately obtained as soon after exposure as is possible. If the pregnant woman has any positive rubella antibody titer, nothing further need be done. If the titer is negative, proceed.
2. Administer 15 to 20 ml of IG, observing the usual precautions for administration of such large doses.
3. Inform the patient as to the unpredictable result prior to undertaking this form of therapy. Of course, this method should be used only when therapeutic abortion will not be considered.

If IG is used in rubella prophylaxis, the titer should always be repeated. A persistently negative titer indicates that infection has not occurred and will be an indication for live rubella virus vaccine once pregnancy is ended. *A positive titer* developing in an initially seronegative woman who has received IG is *indicative of infection* and not passive acquisition of antibody. The parents should be informed of this fact and appropriate action taken, if indicated.

OTHER USES FOR IMMUNE GLOBULIN

A variety of conditions, circumstances, and diseases have occasioned attempts at IG prophylaxis. In many of these circumstances, the outcome is simply unknown and uncertain, and little harm is done save for the cost and discomfort of administering IG. In others, more appropriate therapy may be delayed or displaced by the erroneous belief that IG will be effective. In a few cases, IG is contraindicated and prophylaxis should not be attempted because there is clear-cut evidence of lack of effectiveness and a small risk of adverse consequences. The following are common circumstances under which IG has been considered or used.

THE PREMATURE INFANT

Many premature infants are susceptible to serious bacterial and viral infections during early life. Because these infants have not received the usual amount of transplacental antibody, it was considered theoretically possible to supply IG antibody passively and to thus protect them against significant infection. There is no conclusive evidence that administering IG will be of any benefit to prematurely born infants, and its use is not recommended.

ASTHMA AND OTHER ALLERGIC DISEASES

Often, the frustration of repetitive or continuous asthma, or a serious allergic disorder in other organs, compels the physician to seek any possible remedy, including single or repetitive doses of IG. There is absolutely no evidence that a patient with asthma or any allergic disorder benefits from IG. Its use in these conditions is futile and should not be undertaken. One abuse of IG is its intradermal administration to asthmatic patients. There is no indication for such use and the evidence offered is insubstantial and inadequate to recommend this application of IG.

THE CHILD WITH REPETITIVE INFECTIONS

If a child has repetitive infectious episodes or seemingly infectious episodes (such as those that occur with allergic rhinitis) and no demonstrable defect in IG or antibody synthesis, then the administration of IG is not indicated. In fact, a large number of studies clearly indicate that no benefit can be expected from such administration. This area represents the largest abuse of IG. In the frustrating circumstance of a child appearing repetitively in the office with relatively minor upper respiratory tract infections, both physician and mother desire some magic remedy. Often, IG is selected and if by chance the child's infectious pattern temporarily diminishes concomitant with the administration of IG, the physician, the parent, and even the patient may have an almost mystical and religious conviction of its effectiveness. I have had the repeated experience that following thorough immunologic investigation of individuals in this circumstance, with no convincing evidence for antibody deficiency, parents and physicians absolutely refuse to halt IG administration. I have had parents stomp angrily from the consultation room when discontinuation of IG was recommended, despite the fact that several controlled studies have clearly indicated that IG is of no benefit to such patients.

SINGLE SEVERE BACTERIAL, VIRAL, OR FUNGAL INFECTIONS

Often in a desperate clinical situation involving a life-threatening or very severe infectious disease, the clinician is tempted to add IG to the usual therapy in an effort to turn the tide in favor of the patient. There are many anecdotal reports of favorable outcomes in such life-threatening situations when IG was added to more standard therapy. The difficulty with each of these reports is that numerous forms of therapy were being used and attributing the beneficial effect to IG is no more than temporal and discounts the continuous effect of all other treatment. Unfortunately, controlled studies are unavailable and often impossible in such circumstances because each patient represents his own experiment. It is difficult to conceive that IG could be beneficial in such episodes; however, it is equally difficult to disprove its value. There is some experimental evidence in carefully controlled infections in animals that homologous serum antibody can ameliorate the effects of artificially induced infection, particularly when used in conjunction with appropriate antibiotics. However, these are laboratory-controlled circumstances in which the dose and timing of both infection and antibody administration are optimal, conditions that are impossible to duplicate in cases of clinical infectious disease. Frequently, the best effect is observed in animals receiving antibody *prior* to infection.

Most infectious disease and immunologic experts do not believe that IG has a role in such isolated episodes of infection and in an otherwise healthy host. In one situation, IG administration may be indicated. Patients with thermal burns are susceptible to pseudomonas and staphylococcal infections. Results of attempts to reduce the pseudomonas component through IG administration have varied. Experimental approaches have used specific high titered pseudomonas serum and globulins in experimental models, with demonstrable benefit. Additionally, animal studies have demonstrated that passive antibody can influence the outcome of staphylococcal and pseudomonas infections if administered shortly before, or concomitant with, infection. In the burned patient, such benefit may, in fact, occur. The burn is initially contaminated but active infection has not yet taken place. Thus it is possible that if an appropriate amount of antibody can be delivered, such patients might benefit by reduction of pseudomonas infections (and possibly staphylococcal infections). Administering IG might be useful because antibiotic therapy is often unsuccessful and such patients may succumb to septicemia. An additional reason for using IG is the subtle immunologic change that occurs in burned patients which can result in deficient antibody synthesis and distribution. As a result, many experts recommend large doses of IG (in the range of 1 ml/kg for three or four doses during the first week of burn treatment). There are neither standard guidelines nor universally accepted regimens or dosages. The one suggested above did result in some benefit in a single study, and is recommended to those who wish to employ IG in these situations.

THE MALNOURISHED OR "FAILURE TO THRIVE" INFANT

Malnourished infants and those who fail to thrive are given IG in the mistaken notion that they are deficient and that this will somehow assist in both increasing their nutritional status and in preventing infection. There is no evidence that IG is of any benefit to patients in either group unless there is a demonstrable immunoglobulin–antibody defect. Most of these children do not have this type of defect and do not need IG.

REFERENCES

Beasley RP, Stevens CE: Vertical transmission of HBV and interruption with globulin. In Vyas GN (ed): Viral Hepatitis. Philadelphia, Franklin Institute Press, 1978

Bellanti J (ed): Immunology II. Philadelphia, WB Saunders, 1979

Brunell PA, Gershon AA: Passive immunization against varicella-zoster infections. J Infect Dis 127:415–418, 1973

Ellis EF, Henney CS: Adverse reactions following administration of human gamma globulin. J Allergy 43:45–50, 1969

Haeney MR, Carter GF, Yeoman WB et al: Long-term parenteral exposure to mercury in patients with hypogammaglobulinemia. Br Med J 2:12–14, 1979

Krugman S et al: Viral hepatitis, type B studies on the natural history and prevention re-examined. New Engl J Med 300:101–105, 1979

Krugman S, Ward R, Giles JP et al: Infectious hepatitis: Studies on the effectiveness of gamma globulin and on the incidence of inapparent infections. JAMA 174:823–826, 1960

Matheson DS, Clarkson TW, Gelfand EW: Mercury toxicity (acrodynia) induced by long-term injection of gamma globulin. J Pediatr 97:153–155, 1980

Maynard JE: Passive immunization against hepatitis B: A review of recent studies and comments on current aspects of control. Am J Epidemiol 107:77–86, 1978

Medical Research Council Working Party: Hypogammaglobulinemia in the United Kingdom. Lancet 1:163–166, 1969

Ross AH: Modification of chickenpox in family contacts by administration of gamma globulin. New Engl J Med 267:369–373, 1962

Stiehm ER: Standard and special human immune serum globulins as therapeutic agents. Pediatrics 63:301–319, 1979 (Note: This report contains an exhaustive and detailed list of references.)

Stiehm ER, Fudenberg HH: Antibodies to gamma globulin in infants and children exposed to isologous gamma globulin. Pediatrics 35:229–234, 1965

Stiehm ER, Fulginiti VA (eds): Immunologic Disorders in Infants and Children. Philadelphia, WB Saunders, 1980

Stokes J Jr, Maris EP, Gellis SS: Chemical, clinical and immunological studies on the products of human plasma fractionation. XI. The use of concentrated normal human serum in the prophylaxis and treatment of measles. J Clin Invest 23:531–540, 1944

Vyas GH, Perkins HA, Fudenberg HH: Anaphylactoid transfusion reactions associated with anti-IgA. Lancet 2:312–313, 1968

24

Special Immune Globulins

Vincent A. Fulginiti

The pharmacology and all biologic characteristics of special immune globulins (SIG) do not differ from those described in Chapter 23 for immune globulin (IG). The only significant difference between these preparations and IG is in the specific antibody content. In most instances, the SIGs are collected from donors who are either known to have specific antibody titers against an infectious agent or who have been stimulated with a vaccine to evoke such specific antibody. The value of SIGs lies in their use for specific disease prevention. In some cases, they improve upon the effectiveness of IG, and in others, they are effective when IG is not. All SIGs are labeled by the disease for which they are intended to be used in prophylaxis or treatment.

RABIES IMMUNE GLOBULIN

Passive antibody has been used in the prophylaxis against rabies since the late 19th century. However, the lack of vaccines that were 100% effective, combined with experimental evidence that rabies virus replication might be inhibited during the early incubation period by passive antibody suggested that this modality could be added to vaccine prophylaxis on a more regular basis. Support for the use of passive antibodies was derived from a unique experience in Iran, in which a rabid wolf bit 27 persons, more than half of whom had bites on the head or neck. Three of these persons were treated with vaccine alone and all died from rabies; one of seven who received vaccine and a single dose of antirabies serum died from the disease; and there were no deaths among the five who received both vaccine and two doses of antirabies serum.

The serum was of equine origin and was the only product available at the time. In the early 1970s, a specific rabies immune globulin (RIG) was developed, prepared from donors with high antibody titers stimulated by vaccine.

Rabies immune globulin of human origin has several distinct advantages over that of equine origin. First, it is unassociated with significant serious sensitivity side-effects such as commonly occur with exposure to horse antigens. Second, because it is of human origin, it is removed from the circulation at a slower pace (see Chapter 23) and hence has a more prolonged effect. Because it is always used simultaneously with vaccine, exact dosage recommendations have undergone several modifications. Early on, large doses were associated with significant suppression of the antibody-stimulating capacity of the vaccine; hence, the currently recommended dose of 20 IU/kg of body weight has been arrived at as an effective compromise between immune suppression and adequate provision of antirabies antibody.

Rabies immune globulin is administered as soon after exposure as is possible and usually concomitant with the first does of rabies vaccine. For specific indications for its use, see Chapter 15 on rabies.

Rabies immune globulin is supplied in 2-ml and 10-ml vials that contain 150 IU/ml. All the precautions for administering IG that were indicated in Chapter 23 should be followed for the administration of RIG.

VARICELLA-ZOSTER IMMUNE GLOBULIN

As indicated in Chapter 23, varicella has been modified by large doses of IG. However, varicella has not been prevented, even following administration of very large doses. Philip Brunell and co-workers first developed zoster immune globulin (ZIG), using donors who had antibody titers against varicella of 1:256 or higher. Most often, these were persons who had recently experienced zoster, because this recrudescence of varicella was associated with an anamnestic antibody response. More recently, varicella zoster immune globulin (VZIG) has been prepared and is licensed and distributed commercially. It can be obtained by calling consultants at regional American Red Cross Blood Banks. Current lots of VZIG have antibody titers in the range of 1:1024 to 1:2048 as measured by the FAMA (fluorescent antibody to membrane antigens) test.

Varicella-zoster immune globulin should be administered to patients at high risk for developing progressive varicella. It is not to be used in healthy children. The following are considered candidates for VZIG if exposure to varicella has occurred: (1) patients with leukemia or lymphoma; (2) patients with congenital or acquired immunodeficiency of any type; and (3) patients receiving immunosuppressive medication likely to induce susceptibility to serious varicella. In general, this necessitates using drugs that suppress cell-mediated immune (CMI) function such as occurs with the use of 2 mg/kg/day of prednisone.

Children in these categories should be considered candidates for VZIG if exposure has occurred under the following circumstances: (1) intimate household contact, usually with a sibling or with another person residing in the patient's home or; (2) prolonged contact with a playmate or hospital patient. The judgment as to the extent of contact is usually based on time and is necessarily arbitrary. Varicella is highly contagious and if there has been more than 1 hour of contact with a person with the disease, the susceptible individual should receive VZIG.

Any patient with a negative or unknown history for varicella prior to contact should be considered a candidate. Children less than 15 years old should always be considered candidates.

If used, VZIG should be administered within 96 hours after exposure. It is clear from the experimental studies thus far that the sooner after exposure VZIG is administered, the more effective it is in preventing or ameliorating subsequent disease. There is some dispute as to whether VZIG should be administered at any time after exposure but ordinarily it will not be recommended if exposure occurred more than 96 hours previously.

One sometimes controversial indication for VZIG is that involving the newborn whose mother has varicella. Gershon's studies suggest that an infant born to a mother with varicella has a high risk of acquiring severe, even fatal, disease. As a result, the CDC recommends that a newborn whose mother has contracted varicella less than five days before delivery or within 48 hours after delivery be a candidate for immediate VZIG.

The precise dose of VZIG is uncertain. In most previous studies, total volumes of between 3 and 5 ml have been used. Consultation at the time of need will indicate the currently recommended dose.

HEPATITIS B IMMUNE GLOBULIN

In 1977, a potentially significant advance was made in the prophylaxis of hepatitis B infections when gamma globulin containing high titers against hepatitis B virus became available. Hepatitis B immune globulin (HBIG) is prepared from hepatitis-B-antigen-negative donors and resultant antibody titers exceed 1 : 500,000. In contrast, most lots of IG contain 1 : 2 to 1 : 64 levels of antibody against hepatitis B virus. The effectiveness of HBIG has been substantiated in studies of institutionalized children, of persons accidentally exposed to hepatitis B virus containing blood or other body fluids, of renal dialysis patients and of workers in whom hepatitis B represents a special risk. In addition, spouses of patients with hepatitis B have been protected with HBIG. The effectiveness of its use in newborn infants is more controversial; HBIG and IG both appear to influence the incubation period of hepatitis B virus infection in the infant but do not necessarily prevent it.

Hepatitis B immune globulin is an expensive biologic. There is much dispute concerning the interpretation of the effectiveness of HBIG as compared with that of IG, despite the theoretic advantages of the higher titered HBIG. *Tentative recommendations are included here, but the reader is cautioned that future recommendations may vary, based on additional analysis of available data and on accumulation of additional information.*

In so-called "minimal" exposure, such as occurs when there is injury with a contaminated needle or when blood or other infected material is splashed onto a mucosal surface, it is recommended that HBIG be given as soon as possible after exposure. A dose of 0.05 to 0.07 ml/kg should be administered within the first 7 days following exposure and this dose should be repeated 25 to 30 days later. Some experts advise that IG can be used in a similar dose if HBIG is unavailable.

Infants whose mothers are HB virus-positive during the last trimester of pregnancy, whether by infection or by chronic carriage, should receive a single dose of 0.5 to 1.0 ml/kg of HBIG as soon as possible after birth. This dose may be administered to infants up to 48 hours old (if HBIG is unavailable, 0.5 ml/kg of IG can be substituted). It is uncertain at the present writing whether doses should be repeated at monthly intervals (0.16 ml/kg) or simply once at 3 or 6 months of age (see Chapter 23). This is one of the areas likely to undergo change as additional data are received.

A need for HBIG may also be indicated in the following: (1) sexual contacts of persons infected with hepatitis B virus (in general, this should be a continued contact, such as occurs between spouses); (2) those in custodial institutions in which hepatitis B infections have occurred; (3) patients and personnel involved in renal dialysis, where high rates of transmission have been observed.

In general, everyone should be tested for hepatitis B surface antigen, and only those who are negative should receive HBIG. However, timing may be such that prudence dictates the administration of HBIG while the serologic determination is made. In renal dialysis units or in custodial situations, it is worthwhile to retest for anti-hepatitis-B surface antigen antibody at regular intervals (every 3 to 4 months) in order to detect seroconversion. When this occurs, future doses of HBIG need not be administered.

Some experts recommend that large doses of HBIG (0.5 ml/kg of body weight) be given to those who receive contaminated blood transfusions. This is a very controversial indication and the usefulness of HBIG is uncertain.

Administration of HBIG is not indicated for clinically manifested hepatitis B virus infection. Many physicians prefer to substitute IG for HBIG in certain situations, such as that of personnel in a custodial institution. The rationale here is both in the presumed equivalent effectiveness if larger doses are given, and in the difference in cost and availability of the two products (see Chap. 23 for more complete discussion).

VACCINIA IMMUNE GLOBULIN

Henry Kempe and colleagues have clearly demonstrated the effectiveness of vaccinia immune globulin (VIG) in both the prevention and the treatment of complications of smallpox vaccination and in the prevention of smallpox itself. With the elimination of smallpox world-wide, and the corresponding reduction in smallpox vaccination, this product should find little use in the future. However, since 4 million doses of smallpox vaccine have been administered in the United States in 1980 despite a recommendation by the World Health Organization (WHO) that the product no longer be given to anyone, it is possible that persons will continue to experience complications of vaccination and that VIG will be needed as part of therapy. For this reason, a description of the product is contained in this chapter, although it is anticipated that both the indications for its use and the need for manufacturing the product will disappear in the future.

Vaccinia immune globulin is prepared from donors with known antibody content in their plasma. In our laboratories, VIG has been measured at neutralizing antibody levels of 1 : 128 or higher in various lots.

When used prophylactically, VIG is administered concomitantly with smallpox vaccination and to those persons likely to experience complications. For example, in the past, eczematous children who needed smallpox vaccinations because of travel to smallpox-endemic areas were given VIG in a dose of 0.3 ml/kg of body weight. Similarly, pregnant women who needed vaccinations received an identical dose.

Following smallpox vaccination, a variety of complications arise which can be treated with VIG alone. Accidental auto-inoculation involving eczematoid skin or single or multiple sites in normal skin may be effectively treated with 0.6 ml/kg of VIG. Auto-inoculation of the eye, however, represents a contraindication to VIG administration, because an adverse immunologic consequence (clouding of the cornea) has been observed in those so treated.

More serious complications of vaccinations such as vaccinia necrosum (progressive vaccinia) necessitate both the administration of large doses of VIG and antiviral chemotherapy and immunologic measures. In these situations, the dose of VIG is determined primarily by biologic events and by measurement in the patient. Often, a dose as high as 1 to 10 ml/kg over time has been used. Children with these complications should be treated in large medical centers where facilities for virologic and immunologic diagnosis and treatment are readily available.

Finally, nonimmunized persons who are exposed to smallpox may be given VIG in order to prevent or modify the natural disease. A dose of 0.3 ml/kg has been used and smallpox vaccine has been administered simultaneously.

MUMPS IMMUNE GLOBULIN AND PERTUSSIS IMMUNE GLOBULIN

In the past, both of these products were available and used despite extensive reports indicating that they had little or no effect. In 1980, they were removed from commercial distribution in the United States and hence are not considered further here.

TETANUS IMMUNE GLOBULIN

Since tetanus is primarily a toxic disease, the use of passive antibody following potential inoculation of *Clostridia tetani* was commonplace. The theoretic premise on which this treatment was based resulted in both effective prophylaxis and partial treatment of clinical tetanus. One significant detraction to the use of serum prophylaxis was the occurrence of horse serum sensitivity in recipients. Significant anaphylactic and serum sickness reactions occurred, severely limiting or complicating the use of tetanus antitoxin. Tetanus immune globulin (TIG) became generally available in the early 1970s. Since that time, it has effectively replaced tetanus antitoxin of equine origin in the management of tetanus-prone injuries and in the treatment of tetanus.

Nonimmunized persons sustaining tetanus-prone injuries should be given 250 to 500 IU of TIG by the intramuscular route. Treatment of clinical tetanus will necessitate doses of TIG in excess of 3000 units (see Chap. 8 on tetanus).

ANTI-D-IMMUNE-GLOBULIN (ANTI-RH$_0$) IMMUNE GLOBULIN (RhIG)

Anti-Rh$_0$ immune globulin (RhIG) is a high-titer globulin directed against the major rhesus antigen present on human erythrocytes. RhIG use is indicated in an Rh-negative mother who is also D$_u$-negative, provided the mother has not already been sensitized to the Rh factor. RhIG is given to the mother, never to the infant. It is generally administered as soon after birth as possible, under the following conditions: the infant should be Rh-negative or D_u-positive, and should have a negative Coomb's test or positive test caused by antibodies other than those to D antigen. The above indications apply to term deliveries.

Miscarriages, abortions, or ectopic pregnancies may also sensitize mothers to D antigen. RhIG should be given to Rh-negative nonsensitized women in these circumstances within 72 hours of delivery of the products of conception.

If by accident Rh-positive blood is transfused into an Rh_o D_u-negative individual, RhIG can be given in order to prevent Rh sensitization.

The dose of RhIG is 1 ml given intramuscularly. If there has been a large exchange of blood between the fetus and the mother, an additional dose may be needed. In mismatched blood transfusions, the amount of RhIG is dependent upon the volume of packed Rh-positive cells infused; 1 ml is given for each 15 ml of blood infused.

Recently, the American College of Obstetricians and Gynecologists considered a recommendation that all pregnant Rh-negative women be given RhIG at 28 weeks gestation in order to prevent antepartum immunization in the third trimester. They decided not to accept this recommendation, but it is apparent that individual physicians may wish to consider it. A number of experts believe that this would be excessive use of RhIG and that it would result in as many as 100 unnecessary injections of RhIG for every case in which antepartum immunization might occur.

Some consider amniocentesis results a basis for determining whether to use RhIG in the Rh-negative pregnant woman. In addition, it has been recommended that in cases of massive fetal-maternal hemorrhaging, titered amounts of RhIG rather than the usual 1-ml dose should be given. The suggestion has been made that 10 μ of RhIG for every milliliter of estimated fetal blood transferred to the maternal circulation be used.

REFERENCES

Blake PA, Feldman RA, Buchanan TM et al: Serologic therapy of tetanus in the United States. JAMA 235:42–45, 1976

Brunell PA, Ross A, Miller LH et al: Prevention of varicella by zoster immune globulins. New Engl J Med 280:1191–1194, 1969

Davey MG, Zipursky A: McMaster conference on prevention of Rh immunization. Vox Sang 36:50–64, 1979

Freda VJ, Gorman JG, Pollack W et al: Prevention of Rh hemolytic disease—ten years experience with Rh immune globulin. New Engl J Med 292:1014–1018, 1975

Fulginiti VA: Poxvirus diseases. In Kelley VC, Brennemann R (ed): Practice of Pediatrics. Hagerstown, Harper & Row, 1981

Gershon AA, Steinberg S, Brunell PA: Zoster immune globulin: A further assessment. New Engl J Med 290:243–246, 1974

Habel K, Koprowski H: Laboratory data supporting the clinical trial of antirabies serum in persons bitten by a rabid wolf. Bull WHO 13:773–780, 1955

Kempe CH: Studies on smallpox and complications of smallpox vaccination. Pediatrics 26:176–182, 1960

Kempe CH, Bowles C, Meikeljohn G et al: The use of vaccinia immune globulin in the prophylaxis of smallpox. Bull WHO 25:41–47, 1961

Kohler PF, Dubois RS, Merrill DA et al: Prevention of chronic neonatal hepatitis B infection with antibody to the hepatitis B surface antigen. New Engl J Med 291:1378–1381, 1974

Krugman S, Giles JP, Hammond J: Viral hepatitis, type B (MS-2 strain): Prevention with specific hepatitis B immune serum globulin. JAMA 218:1665–1667, 1971

Loofbourow JC, Cabasso VJ, Roby RE et al: Rabies immune globulin (human): Clinical trials and dose determinations. JAMA 217:1825–1828, 1971

Rubbo SD, Suri JC: Passive immunization against tetanus with human immune globulin. Br Med J 2:79–80, 1962

Sikes RK: Human rabies immune globulin. Publ Health Rep 84:797, 1969

Stiehm ER: Standard and special human immune serum globulins as therapeutic agents. Pediatrics 63:301–319, 1979

Szmuness W, Prince AM, Goodman M et al: Hepatitis B immune serum globulin in prevention of non-parenterally transmitted hepatitis B. New Engl J Med 290:701–705, 1974

25
Vaccines in Development

Vincent A. Fulginiti

The development of new vaccines represents an advancement of technology, of science, and of practical medicine. A single accomplishment in any of these areas is usually not sufficient to guarantee a useful product. Often, antigens can be isolated, packaged, and tested in animals but prove to be of little use, because they afford humans little or no protection or are unsafe. Conversely, we may discover the principle of protection as a result of scientific investigation only to be stymied by technologic hurdles in the manufacture of a usable vaccine. And, on some occasions, science and technology combine to produce a theoretically useful product that is found to have practical limitations in its application. Vaccines previously discussed in this text have met all of these requirements and, as a result, are in common usage. The vaccines and biologics discussed in this review will represent various stages of development in the spectrum from science to application.

Some of the vaccines and biologics to be discussed will become part of everyday practice; the use of others will be indefinitely delayed, and still others will fall by the wayside, an interesting footnote in the historic search for prevention of infectious diseases. All are of interest to us because they represent incremental steps in the improvement of child health, whatever the outcome.

VIRUS VACCINES

VARICELLA VACCINE

Chicken pox is an infectious childhood disease of low to moderate morbidity and negligible mortality in the healthy child. Even at best, it represents an unpleasant interlude in a child's life. For a small group of children and for some adults, varicella may be serious, severe, and life-threatening. Those with immunologic deficiencies secondary to disease or to administration of immunosuppressive therapy may experience severe primary varicella with visceral involvement. In addition, those who have had varicella prior to development of an immunosuppressing disease may, on receipt of immunosuppressive therapy, have their varicella virus rekindled from its latent site with migration to the skin and production of the zoster form of illness.

Protection against varicella is desirable, but the biology of and the immunologic response to the virus pose significant problems and difficulties in developing strategies for control. Among the difficulties encountered are the capacity of the virus to go "underground," that is, to become latent in neuronal cells with the potential for reemergence by transit along nerves to produce cutaneous zoster, and, on occasion, to disseminate severe varicella zoster disease. Latency in human viruses is poorly understood. It is not clear why the virus becomes resident in quiescent form, or what keeps it that way for years or for a lifetime, or why it reemerges in some persons.

On the technical side, varicella virus is so closely bound to human cells that in early virologic work, obtaining a cell-component-free virus preparation was impossible. During the past decade, a group of Japanese workers, led by Dr. Michiaki Takahashi, have successfully cultivated varicella virus in a series of tissue culture transfers and have obtained a vaccine preparation of attenuated live virus (Oka strain) suitable for trials in humans.

Proceeding cautiously, this group of Japanese investigator/clinicians has tested the live varicella virus vaccine (LVV) in successive groups of humans from adults to the target population—groups of children with lymphatic malignancies who are susceptible to the disease. What follows is a summary of their results to date and prospects for the future.

Initially, a small group of healthy, home-living children were given the vaccine. Of 18 susceptible children exposed to varicella, none became ill with chicken pox, and neutralizing antibodies developed in all following administration of LVV. The expected attack rate for varicella is approximately 87%. Dr. Takahashi and his colleagues have reported a near 100% attack rate among 19 children in similar circumstances to the vaccine recipients but living in different homes.

Children at high risk for increased varicella morbidity and mortality were the next recipients of LVV. In sequence, children with steroid-treated nephrosis and with leukemia and solid tumors received LVV. As a precautionary safety measure, chemotherapy was discontinued one week prior to LVV administration in the group with malignancies. Neutralizing antibodies developed in all children in both groups (26 recipients in all, measured one month post-LVV). In two children in the group with malignancies, a few vescicles developed 2 and 4 weeks after LVV. None of the remaining 24 children had significant symptoms.

More than 500 children in these same categories have now been reported to have received LVV in Japan; a few children with malignancies and a few susceptible adults have been immunized in the United States.

These very preliminary studies support the following conclusions:

1. The vaccine is highly antigenic and neutralizing antibodies develop in most susceptible recipients (95%).
2. Antibody persisted in most of a small group followed for 2½ years.
3. More than 20 recipients were judged to be immune upon exposure to the wild virus as evidenced by lack of development of clinical disease.
4. The vaccine virus appears to be truly attenuated in that no symptoms appeared in healthy children who received it. Fever and numerous papules developed in many recipients who were immunocompromised, but without serious consequences.
5. It is too soon to comment on latency and the occurrence of zoster.

In the United States, controversy concerning the use of varicella vaccine has been evident. Protagonists for its use cite the Japanese experience as evidence that theoretic risks have not been realized. Further, they point out the benefit of active immunization for high-risk patients, as opposed to the random use of passive antibody for each exposure (see Chap. 23 and 24).

Antagonists to varicella immunization cite continuing theoretic concerns, asking such questions as: Will zoster develop more often and be more severe in LVV recipients? Will injection of attenuated virus alter the potential for latency and reactivation? Will peripheral nerves be exposed to vaccine virus more readily and enhance entry into the sites of latency? Is there an age-related latency potential? Will early administration of LVV enhance this potential? Will infant immunization displace varicella into adolescence and adult life, when the disease is more serious? What is the actual risk-to-benefit ratio for such a mild disease in healthy persons?

There is much debate and argument and counterargument with little resolution at present. What is certain is that cautious but progressive trials are under way, principally in high-risk patients. It is too soon to predict the outcome of these investigations in terms of ordinary medical practice. I can conceive of a situation in which LVV may become available for highly selective groups of children and for adult patients in high-risk circumstances. It is unlikely that LVV will soon be made available for routine use in healthy infants and children. The latter use will depend upon adequate demonstration of almost absolute safety and effectiveness in that the disease to be prevented is ordinarily mild and without substantial risk.

OTHER HERPES VIRUS VACCINES

Concomitant with the development of LVV, interest continues in vaccines against some very common related viruses—herpes simplex, cytomegalovirus (CMV), and Epstein-Barr virus (EBV). These are all members of the DNA herpes virus group and have many common characteristics, including the potential for latency and reemergence months to years after the primary infection. We will not review the biology of each of these agents separately but simply consider the status of vaccine development. The reader should consider that the controversy and questions asked concerning live varicella virus vaccine apply, to some degree, to each of these other herpes viruses.

Congenital cytomegalovirus infections probably affect 1% of all newborn infants. Prolonged observation has suggested that CMV is a major cause of mental retardation, hearing loss, and recrudescent infections in immunosuppressed persons. However, both the biology and the epidemiology of CMV are not fully understood. Despite significant advances in these areas, many basic questions remain unanswered. In 1974, British investigators reported the isolation and adaptation of a strain of CMV (AD 169) in human embryo and human foreskin fibroblasts. Medical students and laboratory workers voluntarily received this tissue-culture-grown CMV by the oral, intradermal, or subcutaneous route. Subcutaneous inoculation appeared to be antigenic in almost all of the volunteers tested. The complement-fixing antibody initially detected persisted for one year. No virus was detected in bodily secretions and no significant adverse effects were observed.

In the United States, a different CMV isolate was adapted to human diploid embryonic lung cells at the Wistar Institute. Plotkin and his colleagues developed a final virus preparation known as Towne-125 which was then subjected to extensive and exhaustive safety tests in animals and in tissue culture systems. These studies showed no evidence of adverse effects, including oncogenicity. The Wistar group then undertook cautious initial trials of human immunization. Subcutaneous inoculation again proved the material to be antigenic, and both antibody and cell-mediated immunity (CMI) responses were detectable within 2 weeks after the vaccine had been received. As in the British studies, virus was not recovered from various body sites, and no transmission from vaccine recipients to exposed susceptible contacts was observed. Although no adverse systemic reactions were apparent, local reactions at the site of inoculation occurred approximately at the same time the immunologic response was noted. These reactions appeared to be trivial.

These investigations with CMV immunization have polarized the medical community. Many responsible physicians and scientists do not feel that human immunization should proceed until critical questions concerning the biology and epidemiology of CMV infections are better understood. Questions of latency, of the precise immunologic response that results in immunity, and of safety have been raised. Yet equally responsible physicians and scientists advocate cautious investigation of CMV vaccine because of the predictable toll the virus takes, as was outlined. Its very ubiquitousness argues for exploration of prophylaxis, according to the protagonists.

Studies have continued amid this controversy. The Towne-125 agent was given to 12 sero-negative adult patients who were candidates for renal transplants. The immunologic findings for these persons did not differ from those of the prior studies. Following transplant, half the recipients shed cytomegalovirus upon receiving immunosuppressive therapy. Biologic markers suggested that the virus shed differed from the vaccine strain. Some experts have concluded that immunization with the Towne-125 strain does not prevent reinfection with different strains of CMV. Even the results of this study among the 12 vaccine recipients point out the difficulties to be encountered in evaluating vaccine effect when so much remains to be learned about the basic characteristics of the infection in nature. I believe that CMV immunization should be reserved until the immunologic and virologic characteristics of the natural infection are more fully understood.

Herpes simplex viruses are among the most ubiquitous and prevalent of all infectious agents. Diseases caused by herpesvirus range from the uncomfortable (herpes stomatitis) to the life-threatening (herpes encephalitis). Many of the problems of the biology and immunology of this group of DNA viruses are shared by herpes simplex viruses and will not be reviewed here. Herpesvirus immunization has been used in some experimental animal models for determining the biologic properties of the virus and the immune response. Serious consideration of herpesvirus immunization has been hampered by inadequate knowledge in these areas. I know of one current effort involving the development and cautious testing of a subunit vaccine. Little data are available and many of the same problems encountered for CMV and varicella will need to be addressed before herpesvirus vaccine can be developed and used.

RESPIRATORY VIRUS VACCINES

Influenza

Inactivated influenza vaccines are available and in use as was discussed in Chapter 8. What we will consider here are approaches to solving the several problems encountered in vaccine manufacture, distribution, and use. In Chapter 16, Dr. E. Russell Alexander reviewed the antigenic changes that influenza virus can undergo, sometimes suddenly and with grave consequences secondary to the pandemics that ensue throughout the world's population. Efforts to adapt to the changing antigenicity of influenza virus have been hampered by the following: the interval necessary for identification of the hemagglutinin (H) and neuraminidase (N) structure of the currently prevalent strains; the need to identify laboratory strains that can be adapted for vaccine manufacture; and the time needed to produce the quantities of vaccine necessary for mass immunization efforts. In the swine influenza episode in 1976, all of these difficulties were encountered, and vaccine production was delayed, although finally accomplished. Fortunately, the strain prevalent in Fort Dix did not spread and many experts believe that had it done so, there would have been insufficient time to immunize the population against this variant.

Investigators have turned their attention towards means of altering influenza virus *in vitro* in order to ensure rapid incorporation of the newly identified influenza antigens into a strain that can then undergo massive and rapid replication in pharmaceutical laboratories. If this were accomplished, it might be possible to mass-produce enough vaccine of the appropriate antigenic type to reach the population at risk prior to the natural spread of that virus. Laboratory strategies have included attempts to have influenza viruses transfer genes *in vitro* so that the desired H and N antigens from the current strain can be quickly transferred to the rapidly growing vaccine strain. These attempts at recombinant development offer the likelihood of matching the speed of natural change in influenza virus with that of laboratory adaptation. For example, if a relatively benign attenuated strain of influenza virus could be induced *in vitro* to accept genetic material from a virulent "new" influenza virus, it might be possible, by cloning, to quickly recover a rapidly growing attenuated strain possessing current antigens. This strain could then form the basis of vaccine manufacture, with two possible avenues to pursue. First, the attenuated strain itself might be used as a live, attenuated vaccine. There is a long history of attempts to tame influenza virus in such a fashion so that it provokes active infection in the recipient without producing symptomatology. Combining this approach with the capacity to form recombinants might offer a solution to the changing antigenicity of influenza viruses in nature.

A second alternative would be to mass-produce inactivated vaccines similar to those currently in use but to do so quickly enough and in enough quantity to enable their use prior to epidemic spread.

Another approach to influenza prophylaxis has been the attempt to refine vaccines to eliminate those components of the virus that stimulate undesirable side-effects while preserving those components responsible for evoking appropriate immunologic responses. Techniques such as high-speed zonal ultracentrifigation have contributed to a high degree of purification of influenza viruses. In addition, the facility with which influenza virus can be fragmented into components can be coupled with separation techniques with the result that high-density specific antigen vaccines can be prepared. Mastery of these technologic skills can result in the production of large amounts of type-specific influenza components with which to mass-immunize large populations.

Other approaches are being explored, and undoubtedly new ones will be adapted to vaccine development as investigation of influenza virology and biology continues.

Common Childhood Viruses

For almost two decades, it has been apparent that respiratory syncytial virus, the parainfluenza group of viruses, and selected adenoviruses account for a large proportion of serious respiratory illness in children. Soon after these viruses were discovered and their biologic and epidemiologic properties explored, investigators began to devise strategies for immunization. Initial attempts with adenoviruses were primarily directed toward use in the military, because this group of agents results in much illness in recruits, disrupting their preparation for military service. A fair degree of success has been achieved with such inactivated vaccines against some adenovirus subtypes, but progress in this area has been hampered by the discovery that some adenoviruses were oncogenic or were contaminated with "fellow travelers"; that is, other virus agents that produced oncogenicity *in vitro* or in laboratory animals. These findings have severely limited the applicability of adenovirus immunology to vaccine development. Despite early exploration of the potential for adenovirus immunization among children, there is virtually no activity in this area at present.

The single most important agent in childhood respiratory disease is respiratory syncytial virus (RSV). It accounts for most instances of viral bronchiolitis and much of pneumonia and other lower tract disease. In the 1960s, vaccines were prepared against RSV that were alum-precipitated and inactivated with formalin. Successively tested in adult patients, in adolescents, and in young children, these vaccines appeared to be capable of stimulating antibody, and larger-scale trials were attempted in susceptible infants. The trials ended disastrously when investigators discovered that some young infants who had received RSV-inactivated vaccine developed heightened susceptibilities to the natural virus, resulting in severe bronchiolitis that occasionally was lethal.

Since these early efforts, there has been considerable study of the immunology and epidemiology of RSV infections in children. It seems clear that antibody production alone is not responsible for protection. The role of CMI has recently been delineated, and appears to be a major influence in recovery from, and resistance to, reinfection with respiratory syncytial virus. The interaction between these two components, particularly in early life, is not completely understood. It appears to some, including myself, that increased CMI as a result of receipt of the previously used RSV vaccines, may have resulted in the increased susceptibility to the natural virus.

As further biologic and immunologic characteristics of RSV infection are being worked out, attempts are being made to develop alternative approaches to vaccine development. The most recent of these is consideration of attenuated, live RSV strains as candidates for vaccines that can be applied topically to the respiratory mucosa. Use of a temperature-sensitive mutant (ts-1) has been cautiously investigated but application to sero-negative infants and children has often resulted in undesirable symptomatology. In those who received ts-1 immunization by the respiratory route, afebrile rhinorrhea developed, and a few patients shed virus from the respiratory tract that appeared to revert back to temperature insensitivity. There is now an ongoing search for other mutant viruses with which the desired end of adequate immunization without side-effects might be achieved. Investigators in this area have been buoyed by the fact that with ts-1, they came very close to achieving these objectives.

Parainfluenza virus immunization has been equally unsuccessful when an inactivated vaccine has been used. Although it stimulates serum antibody, no protection is afforded the recipients. In this group of viruses, the lack of effectiveness of immunization is believed to be due to the lack of development of topical IgA antibody. Experimental evidence suggests that the presence of such local antibody may be critical in resisting challenge with virulent virus. As a result, current efforts are directed toward developing an attenuated strain of virus that can be applied directly onto the respiratory mucosa.

Other respiratory agents that produce disease in children and in adult patients are also candidates for virus development. This subject will not be explored further except to note that more than 100 different agents have been indicated in the various viral respiratory syndromes. At one time, Dr. Jonas Salk visualized a day when all or most of these agents would be incorporated in a single vaccine to be administered to young infants, protecting them against the common respiratory infections. We appear to be a long way from realizing this particular dream.

HEPATITIS VIRUS VACCINE

The majority of children are free of overt viral hepatitis throughout childhood. Although many are infected, a large portion experience asymptomatic infection or anicteric mild illness. Most of these children are infected with hepatitis A virus (HAV). Hepatitis B virus (HBV) or non-A non-B hepatitis virus (NANB) infects few children in the United States (see Fig. 25-1).

Selective groups of children, adolescents, and adult patients are at increased risk of symptomatic, even severe, viral hepatitis. Infants born to HBV carriers or to recently infected mothers, children who need frequent blood or blood product transfusions (HBV or NANB), and children with immunodeficiencies are all subject to increased risk of viral hepatitis. Adolescents who abuse drugs, particularly by the intravenous route, may be at increased risk because of their life-style, or because of contamination of intravenous drugs or injection apparatus. Homosexual males also appear to be at increased risk.

Attempts to control hepatitis in the past have focused on supplying sufficient amounts of appropriate antibody in the form of gamma globulin to persons known to be exposed to one of the hepatitis viruses. This approach has been detailed in Chapters 23 and 24. There are obvious shortcomings to passive immunization, in that exposure must be known, the risk must be appreciated by patient and physician, the prophylaxis must be administered early enough, and the gamma globulin must contain the appropriate antibody at a level sufficient to influence disease expression or severity. In addition, some persons experience repetitive exposures, and the repeated use of prophylaxis is both inconvenient and costly. Because of these shortcomings, the search has proceeded for an active immunization method that will confer immunity prior to anticipated exposure and last through all subsequent exposures.

Development of such vaccines has been hampered by imperfect knowledge of the biology and immunology of the hepatitis viruses, by unanswered questions concerning the pathogenesis of the diseases, and by uncertainties in interpretation of early attempts at protection. As knowledge has increased with consistent and painstaking investigation, many of the problems have been overcome. Technologic difficulties have also been overcome, and the prospect for developing effective hepatitis vaccines is at hand.

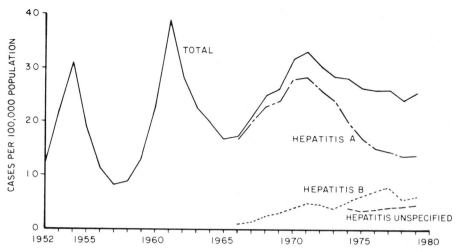

Fig. 25-1. Hepatitis: reported case rates by year, United States, 1952–1979. Viral hepatitis continues to be one of the 5 most frequently reported infectious diseases in the United States. The total number of viral hepatitis cases reported for 1979, although higher than that for 1978, was nearly equal to the numbers reported for 1975 through 1977. Increases were observed in 1979 in the case rates and in the number of cases of all 3 hepatitis types; the largest increase occurred in the unspecified hepatitis category. Persons from 15 through 29 years of age continue to be the group most affected by hepatitis. (Center for Disease Control. Morb Mort Week Rep, 28:54, 1980 [Annual Summary 1979])

It is beyond the scope of this chapter to completely detail the development of hepatitis vaccines. We will give a brief synopsis here, and refer the interested reader to the references for more complete description.

There are large amounts of hepatitis B surface antigen (HBsAg) in the circulation of infected persons, both on an acute and a chronic basis. Hepatitis B vaccines currently under investigation are manufactured by concentration and purification of HBsAg obtained from humans with this antigen in their blood. Both whole viruses and purified polypeptides derived from this source have been used. Animal studies have been limited to investigation in the chimpanzee and have provided initial evidence of antigenicity and safety. All vaccines to date are inactivated by heating or by formalin treatment, or by both. Hepatitis B virus infectivity appears not to be present in any of the lots of the vaccines used in clinical trials. A variety of vaccines have been prepared and are in clinical testing. Most consist of highly concentrated and purified preparations of the 22 nanometer HBsAg particles.

Initial trials were designed to demonstrate the safety of single doses of several of the vaccines. No evidence for active infection or other untoward consequences was observed in volunteers for 6 months or more after administration of the inactivated surface antigen vaccines. Initial antigenic results were somewhat disappointing. An antibody against surface antigen developed to low titers and very slowly, as long as 10 to 14 weeks after immunization. Further purification of the vaccines improved the antigenicity such that antibody was detected in more than 90% of those given two doses. Use of an alum adjuvant improved both the rate and development of serum antibody.

After the initial safety and antigenicity trials, larger scale administration trials were conducted, first among high-risk patients, and then in broader groups. Usually, two to three doses of vaccine at monthly intervals with booster doses a year later were used. Sufficient antigenicity and effectiveness were demonstrated, encouraging further trials in which it is anticipated that the vaccine's usefulness will be established.

Total control of hepatitis B seems impractical, because the source of vaccine is a limited number of human donors. Therefore, it is likely that initial recommendations will be limited to high-risk groups, including renal dialysis patients, patients who need repetitive blood transfusions, medical personnel dealing with blood and blood products and who are likely to become infected, and so forth.

One unique approach to hepatitis B immunization is the possibility of using bacteria to produce HBsAg by the techniques of DNA recombination and cloning. If this method becomes technically possible and feasible, then the major limitation to vaccine production—the use of human donors—would be obviated, and enough vaccine could be produced to consider global use. The development of HBV vaccine has differed sharply from that of all other viral vaccines. The agent has not been successfully cultivated in an *in vitro* tissue culture system, as has been accomplished for all other viral vaccines. Should this technical hurdle be overcome, the entire vaccine development for hepatitis B would change dramatically.

HAV immunization research, on the other hand, has not reached the same level of activity, and the agent for NANB has not been clearly identified.

VIRAL GASTROENTERITIS VACCINE

A limited number of viral agents appear to be responsible for much of the viral gastroenteritis in children. One of the major agents producing epidemic disease is rotavirus. Recently, type 2 human rotavirus was successfully adapted to growth in tissue culture, and it now seems possible that a vaccine could be prepared. Prior to use of such a product, much more needs to be learned about the immunologic response to rotavirus infection and other gastroenteritis-producing viruses. Major efforts are now directed toward defining and refining immunologic mechanisms in these surface infections. What little is known has been gained by consideration of the epidemiologic characteristics of these infections, plus limited data on oral feeding of rotavirus type 2 to adult volunteers. It appears that type-specific local IgA antibody in the intestinal tract is correlated with resistance to challenge. Serum antibody appears to be correlated but not primary. Further investigation should result in better definition of these characteristics and possible vaccine development.

OTHER VIRUS VACCINES

A variety of illnesses produced by virus infection might be amenable to immunization. Arboviruses, enteroviruses other than polio, and specific agents like the reoviruses might also become candidates for such an approach. At the present time, activity is sparse in these areas and more attention is being paid to vector control where applicable and to other hygienic measures to control spread of infection, rather than to immunologic prevention. In addition, for some of these agents, there is inadequate information on which to base immunoprophylaxis.

Finally, it should be remembered that not all of the currently available viral vaccines are ideal. Usually, if a vaccine is effective and reasonably safe, further inquiry into alternative methods for immunization either ceases or is diminished in intensity. Nevertheless, it is conceivable that refinements will be made in currently available vaccines based on new information resulting from laboratory or other investigations. This certainly has been true for rubella and rabies virus vaccines, in which new methods of preparation have resulted in highly antigenic and equally safe products that have supplanted their predecessors. Thus, although the currently available biologics are enormously useful, even better vaccines may be routinely used in the future.

BACTERIAL VACCINES

PERTUSSIS VACCINE

The debate concerning the risk-to-benefit ratio for pertussis vaccine and its corresponding disease continues and, at times, intensifies. These considerations have been adequately reviewed in the chapter on pertussis. It is clear that significant advances could be made if a pertussis vaccine conferring significant protection without significant side-effects were developed. The classic approach has been to extract antigens from *Bordatella pertussis* that would be immunogenic but would avoid the undesirable side-effects of whole bacteria. From time to time, such extracted antigens have been developed and do appear to lessen local reactions but not to significantly alter systemic reactions. Currently, one major drug manufacturer in the United States is investigating a newly prepared extracted pertussis vaccine, but final assessment is not yet available.

Other approaches have included attempts to separate bacterial pili from pertussis bacilli as a possible immunizing antigen. Pili are those bacterial structures that project from the bacterial cell surface and that appear to be responsible for adhesion of the bacteria to human cells, among other functions. This effort is so preliminary that no results can be reported. However, pili preparations for other bacteria have suggested that vaccines containing this component might be effective.

We also know that pertussis vaccines contain high levels of endotoxin and of adenylate cyclase. The endotoxin component may be deleterious and may contribute to the production of some of the severe reactions seen after pertussis administration. It may be possible to improve current vaccines by limiting the amount of endotoxin and other harmful constituents.

STREPTOCOCCAL VACCINE

For many years, it has been apparent that an effective and safe streptococcal vaccine directed against group A organisms would prevent a great deal of childhood morbidity and mortality from the primary infection, its pyogenic complications, and its nonpyogenic sequelae. In recent years, the emergence of group B streptococci as a major newborn and early infancy pathogen has also suggested immunization as a possible means for control. Any efforts at the development of streptococcal vaccines have been hampered by the potential for stimulating the very immunologic responses the vaccine is intended to prevent. In addition, group A serotypes are numerous and immunity appears to be type-specific. This factor alone results in technologic difficulty in preparing an adequate vaccine.

Early attempts at streptococcal immunization resulted in antibody production, both against the streptococcus and against the shared proteins in cardiac muscle. In 1969, 21 patients received a partially purified type M-3 vaccine and two cases of acute rheumatic fever occurred; a third recipient probably also developed this disease. Analysis of this experience suggests that multiple injections of this particular vaccine may have predisposed to acute rheumatic fever. Since these attempts, intensive effort has been made to separate the M-protein of streptococci from any cross-reacting elements that might induce antibody to cardiac antigens. At least one such preparation has been made, and initial tests in fewer than 20 adult patients suggest that type-specific antibody is induced, and that the reaction is highly specific to M-protein from the strain of streptococcus used in preparation. Immunologic cross-reactivity with heart tissue has not been demonstrated by a variety of methods. This encouraging preliminary observation suggests that streptococcal control through vaccination might be possible in the future. However, the highly specific nature of the response suggests either that multiple antigens would have to be incorporated, each with the same degree of purity and demonstrated lack of cross-reactivity, or that it may be possible to limit the number of types to those with the greatest potential for producing rheumatic fever in the target population.

During the period of these investigations, a marked change in the epidemiology of rheumatic fever occurred in the United States. It is widely believed that the incidence of this disease has dramatically decreased and that mass immunoprophylaxis to prevent rheumatic fever alone would be insufficient reason to use streptococcal vaccines. On the other hand, in many areas of the world, rheumatic fever remains a major problem and immunization programs would have greater rationale.

PSEUDOMONAS VACCINE

Pseudomonas aeruginosa infections have become increasingly common among certain groups of patients. Burn patients, those needing prolonged respiratory assistance, neonates, and immunologically deficient persons may all be susceptible to severe pseudomonas infections. Results of a large number of animal and human studies have suggested that passively administered antibody with high titer against *P. aeruginosa* has been moderately successful in aborting or ameliorating subsequent pseudomonas infections. Effectiveness appears to be related both to the timing and to the titer of antibody in the administered serum or gamma globulin.

Polyvalent pseudomonas vaccines have been developed, and, based upon the previously successful experience with passive immunoprophylaxis, have been administered to burn patients. Pseudomonas septicemia has been prevented, suggesting that this might be an effective adjunct to therapy. Unfortunately, in some trials, the eradication of pseudomonas as a threat in the burn patient has resulted in the supplanting of that organism with other equally undesirable pathogens. There is little question that continued investigation of immunoprophylaxis against pseudomonas may provide valuable means of immunoprophylaxis for selected high-risk patients.

OTHER BACTERIAL VACCINES

The search for effective vaccines against *Hemophilus influenza* continues despite the disappointing results of initial efforts with a polysaccharide vaccine similar to those developed for pneumococcus and meningogoccus. *H. influenza* type B represents a major bacterial pathogen for the very young infant and successful immunization would significantly alter the morbidity and mortality attendant on these infectious episodes. However, young infants react poorly to polysaccharide antigens in general, and extremely poorly to the polysaccharide antigen prepared from *H. influenza*. This has spurred attempts to identify other antigens or to enhance the antigenicity of the polysaccharide by combination with protein substrates. These efforts are in their preliminary stages and have not yet reached the degree of practical clinical trials. There seems to be little question that this is one of the most important investigative areas in all of immunization research. In addition to providing needed protection in young infants against this particular pathogen, solving the immunologic riddle of poor antigenicity of hemophilus polysaccharide in infants might provide clues that would enable us to prepare more effective vaccines against other common pathogens.

Enteric bacterial pathogens represent a major cause of morbidity and mortality throughout the world. Infections such as cholera, salmonella, shigella, and *Escherichia coli* provide a background of illness in certain childhood populations in the world which result in extreme morbidity and mortality when coupled with other viral and bacterial childhood infections. The usual route of immunoprophylaxis, the development of inactivated vaccines, has resulted in relatively ineffective protection with considerable side-effects. Cholera and salmonella vaccines are among the more reactogenic products and the protection they offer is limited both in scope and duration. Current investigational approaches include the use of oral attenuated strains of these bacteria in an attempt to confer local immunity which would result in resistance to challenge by the naturally occurring bacterial agents. These investigations are extremely promising, but very preliminary at the present time.

Another new idea has occurred as the result of the discovery of cross-reacting antigens in seemingly unrelated organisms. For example, certain types of *E. coli* share antigens with *Haemophilus* sp. and with meningococci. Asymptomatic infection with the K-100 type of *E. coli* stimulates antibody against *H. influenzae* type B. Similarly, K-1 strains of *E. coli* induce antibody cross-reaction with the group B meningococcus. Investigation along this line might someday lead to the realization

of protection against these important pediatric diseases by use of innocuous organisms, thus overcoming the difficulties experienced in current attempts at protection.

GENERAL APPROACHES TO IMPROVING IMMUNIZATIONS

ADJUVANTS

Many antigens evoke insufficient immunologic response when
given in their native state. There have been many attempts to enhance
the antigenicity of such biologics by adding materials that enhance
immunologic responsiveness. Most of these materials are designed to
hold the antigen at the site of administration and to release it slowly.
The concept is to permit prolonged antigenic exposure in order to enable
recruitment of more and more B cells, resulting in a quantitatively
larger immunologic response. There may be other mechanisms operative that also result in enhancement. It is conceivable that adjuvants in
some way potentiate the immunologic cell's capacity to respond to
specific antigens. Recent investigations suggest that the mechanisms of
adjuvant action are much more complex than these simple concepts
suggest. The effect of adjuvants may touch a variety of immunologically
active cells and may result in proliferation, in differentiation, in change
in receptors, in induction of and release of mediators, and even in
tropism of the various wandering cells. It is probably more accurate in
the current decade to speak of adjuvant action as a multifaceted function with varying degrees of complexity.

Classic adjuvants have included aluminum compounds, and these are
discussed in Chapter 2. Some years ago, Maurice Hillemen at Merck
Sharp & Dohme investigated the use of an oil-based adjuvant prepared
from peanut oil that appeared to be a marked improvement over the
previously used mineral oil adjuvants (which had a high degree of side-
effects). Other vegetable oil adjuvants have been developed in an effort
to overcome this limitation of mineral oil. The scientific community has
been concerned that the long-term effects of oil adjuvants are unknown.
Theoretically, long-term irritation could result in undesirable local tissue changes and, as a result, oil adjuvants of various types have found
little use in routine immunizations.

The most encouraging new approach is the development of synthetic
adjuvants of carefully defined structure. Complete description of these
agents is beyond the scope of this chapter. The interested reader is
referred to the contributions by Edelman and colleagues listed in the
references. It is clear that, as we develop more highly purified subunit
particles of infectious agents as candidates for vaccines, we may be

compromising the immunogenicity of the final product. This may occur as a result of the intrinsic adjuvant effect conferred upon the smaller unit antigen when it is part of the entire organism or part of a large fragment of the organism. By separation and isolation, we have lost the advantage of this adjuvant effect, even though we may have gained specificity and reduced side-effects. Thus, the search for new adjuvants is an attempt to replace the natural effect of the organism with a compound that is reasonably safe and nonreactive and that can potentiate the antigenicity of the specified bacterial or viral component.

ALTERNATIVE ROUTES OF IMMUNIZATION

In the discussion on enteric bacterial pathogens above, it was implied that oral immunization may offer some advantages. Additionally, topical immunization for many of the respiratory viral agents appears to more closely approximate the natural route of infection, thereby stimulating a more effective immunologic response in the effort to confer upon the host adequate resistance to infection. Oral polio vaccine (OPV) has already provided us with evidence that this approach is effective. We know that inactivated polio vaccine, while confering adequate immunity against paralytic disease, does not prevent infection with live poliovirus in the respiratory and intestinal tracts. On the other hand, oral administration of live poliovirus results in infection of mucosal cells and adjacent lymphoid tissue with production of specific secretory IgA antibody, and perhaps other immunologic defenses; this results in resistance of these tissues to reinfection with the same type of poliovirus.

It has become relatively commonplace in investigative laboratories to explore routes of immunization other than the parenteral. Mucosal inoculation, either by spray or drops, has been effective in animals and in humans for a variety of viruses and for some bacteria. In the future, the practitioner may be confronted with vaccines other than OPV that are administered by way of the nose, the pharanx, or the gastrointestinal tract. This approach is not without its problems in that even highly attenuated viruses, when administered by the natural route to susceptible infants, may produce undesirable symptoms similar to those of the disease that the vaccine was intended to prevent. A novel idea to overcoming this phenomenon is the possibility of combining the synthetic adjuvants discussed in the foregoing with highly specific antigens from a variety of infectious agents and then to introduce these combinations onto the mucosal surface. It has already been demonstrated that for certain vaccines even the inactivated form, if administered onto the mucosal surface, evokes an antibody response. The effectiveness of this approach has been somewhat limited, but perhaps the inclusion of adjuvants may potentiate the immunogenic effect.

INTRAVENOUS GAMMA GLOBULINS

As discussed partially in Chapter 23, experimental preparations of human gamma globulin are currently being investigated for administration by the intravenous route. Gamma globulin currently available in the United States cannot be administered intravenously because it provokes anaphylactic reactions, owing to the aggregation of immunoglobulin molecules in the concentrated solution. These aggregates are highly anticomplementary and behave as if antigen were present, simulating anaphylaxis in the host. Over the years, numerous attempts have been made to overcome this deficiency of gamma globulin, because intravenous administration would represent a major advantage in both effectiveness and safety. Current methods include acid treatment and various other chemical alterations in the immunoglobulin molecules such that their antibody capacity is retained, but their ability to polymerize is reduced or eliminated. It is anticipated that one or more of these preparations may be commercially available in the near future. Reasonably large-scale trials have been conducted abroad and in the United States and appear to offer useful products for intravenous use in selected circumstances (see Chap. 23 for further discussion).

REFERENCES

Beachey EH, Stollerman GH, Bisno AL: A strep vaccine: How close? Hosp Pract 11:49–57, 1979

Beachey EH et al: Human immune response to immunization with a structurally defined polypeptide fragment of streptococcal M protein. J Exper Med 150:862–874, 1979

Brunell PA: Live attenuated varicella vaccine: Where do we go from here? Hosp Pract 15(9):91–3, 97, 100–101, 1980

Chanock RM, Richardson LS, Belshe RB et al: Prospects for prevention of bronchiolitis caused by respiratory syncytial virus. Pediatr Res 11:264–267, 1977

Conner JS, Speers JF: A comparison between undesirable reactions to extracted pertussis antigen and to whole-cell antigen in DPT combinations. J Iowa Med Soc 53:340–342, 1963

Dudgeon JA: Immunization in times ancient and modern. J Roy Soc Med 73:581–586, 1980

Edelman R, Hardegree MC, Chedid L: Summary of an international symposium on potentiation of the immune response to vaccines. J Infect Dis 141:103–112, 1980

Elek SK, Stern DH: Development of a vaccine against mental retardation caused by cytomegalovirus infection *in utero.* Lancet 1:1–5, 1974

Fulginiti VA, Eller JJ, Sieber OF et al: Respiratory virus immunization. I. A field trial of two inactivated respiratory virus vaccines; an aqueous trivalent parainfluenza virus vaccine and an alum-precipitated respiratory syncytial virus vaccine. Am J Epidemiol 89:435–448, 1969

Gehrz RC, Christianson WR, Linner KM et al: Cytomegalovirus vaccine Arch Intern Med 140:936–939, 1980

Hilleman M, Woodhour AF, Friedman A et al: Studies for safety of adjuvant 65. Ann Allergy 30:477–483, 1972

Issacson RE, Dean EA, Morgan RL et al: Immunization of suckling pigs against enterotoxigenic *Escherichia coli*-induced diarrheal disease by vaccinating dams with purified K99 or 987 P Pili: Antibody production in response to vaccination. Infect Immunol 29:824–826, 1980

Jones RJ, Roe EA, Gupta JL: Controlled trial of pseudomonas immunoglobulin and vaccine in burn patients. Lancet 2:1263–1264, 1980

Katz SL, Klein JO (eds): Prospects for new viral vaccines: A symposium. Rev Infect Dis 2:349–492, 1980 (Note: Includes articles on mucosal vaccination, adjuvants, respiratory syncytial virus, live varicella vaccine, influenza and respiratory viruses prophylaxis, human cell culture rabies vaccine, cytomegalovirus immunization, rotoviruses, and hepatitis B vaccines)

Kempe CH, Gershon AA: Varicella vaccine at the crossroads. Pediatrics 60:930–931, 1977

Lieberman MM, Wright GL, Wolcott KM et al: Polyvalent antisera to pseudomonas ribosomal vaccines: Protection of mice against clinically isolated strains. Infect Immunol 29:489–493, 1980

Marx JL: Vaccinating with bacterial pili. Science 209:1103–1106, 1980

Medearis DN Jr: Human cytomegalovirus immunization prospects. New Engl J Med 296:1289–1290, 1977

Melnick JL: Viral vaccines: New problems and prospects. Hosp Pract 7:104–112, 1978

Melnick JL, Dreesman GR, Hollinger FB: Approaching the control of viral hepatitis type B. J Infect Dis 133:210–228, 1976

Mortimer EA Jr: Pertussis immunization: Problems, perspectives, prospects. Hosp Pract 15(10):103–118, 1980

Ocklitz HW: Vaccinations against bacterial infections. Proc First Int Symp ICP. In Paediatrician 8(s):1:26–36, 1979

Plotkin SA, Brunell PA: Two points of view on herpes virus vaccines. Pediatr 56:494–498, 1975

Price RW, Walz A, Wohlenberg C: Latent infection of sensory ganglia with herpes simplex virus: Efficacy of immunization. Science 188:938–940, 1975

Szmuness W, Stevens CE, Harley ET et al: Hepatitis B vaccine: Demonstration of efficacy in a controlled clinical trial in a high risk population in the United States. N Engl J Med 303:833–841, 1980

Takahashi M, Otsuka T, Okuna Y et al: Live vaccine used to prevent the spread of varicella in children in hospital. Lancet ii:1288–1290, 1974

Tolpin MD, Starr SE, Arbeter AM et al: Inactivated mouse cytomegalovirus vaccine: Preparation, immunogenicity and protective effect. J Infect Dis 142:569–574, 1980

Index

Numerals followed by an "f" indicate a figure; "t" following a page number indicates a table.

Numerous spelling mistakes & misprints. English – split infinitives.
Not sure that typhoid vaccine was that instrumental in
decreasing death rate from typhoid in soldiers or achieved

p.119 – bad misprint immune for susceptible. Sloppy proof-reading

p 120 – SSPE downside but not measles vaccine – see p 124
(possibility of MV → SSPE discussed but not of rv protected against SSPE, & there is evidence that this does affect)

p 121 – First a tuberculin test!!

Pathetically few references – important to verify some of the
more thought-provoking or strange/odd statements that
do occur.

Strongly geared to USA practice

No mention of use of tetanus vaccine in prevention of
neonatal tetanus – prob because now rare in USA but
amazingly short-sighted view.

Annoying habit of referring to work done in text
(eg. Peebles et al on p 100) but not found in references

Chapter on less frequently used vaccines inc. cholera, no
mention of its efficacy

PERTUSSIS – advocates upto 5 y, in certain circumstances 6-7 y, or even re-
for adolescents & adults (p 87)

p.91 by (obvious) friends of the authors are admitted – preliminary unpublished
NCES discussed in one line (no ref given) – but local study done
results quoted. Downside of side effects, std example of wordiness &
superficiality of the book. Details given on p. in numbers.
No mention of efficacy of PV – a burning issue in recent y